Mental Health Care Administration

Mental Health Care Administration

A Guide for Practitioners

Paul Rodenhauser, M.D.
Editor

Ann Arbor
THE UNIVERSITY OF MICHIGAN PRESS

Published in the United States of America by
The University of Michigan Press
Manufactured in the United States of America
⊗ Printed on acid-free paper

2003 2002 2001 2000 4 3 2 1

A CIP catalog record for this book is available from the British Library.

Library of Congress Cataloging-in-Publication Data

Mental health care administration : a guide for
practitioners / Paul Rodenhauser, editor.
p. cm.
Includes bibliographical references and index.
ISBN 0-472-11116-7 (cloth : acid-free paper)
1. Mental health services—Administration. 2. Mental
health services—United States—Administration. I.
Rodenhauser, Paul.
RA790.5.M4185 2000
362.2'068—dc21 99-050531

Preface

My motivation for producing a book on mental health care administration began gathering momentum in 1981. Having just completed the certification examination in administrative psychiatry offered by the American Psychiatric Association (APA), I decided to explore ways to promote interest and expertise in leadership and management among clinicians.

The works of several scholars contributed immensely to my interest in expanding opportunities for education in this field. Milton Greenblatt, Walter Barton, Gail Barton, and Saul Feldman have been most influential. These author-practitioners described and demonstrated ways in which refined and well-focused administrative skills allow certain individuals—as leaders—to affect the treatment of many individuals by embracing the therapeutic environment as a whole.

It has long been recognized that the goals established for mental health care organizations and the therapeutic goals for individuals in need of psychiatric services are intricately interrelated and therefore need to be considered inseparable in the interest of effective outcomes. Clinically informed leadership can enhance the healing environment significantly by facilitating congruence between the organization's mission and the services provided.

My early professional experience included serving as chief resident at the Sheppard and Enoch Pratt Hospital, where Bob Gibson exemplified the combined clinical and leadership expertise required to guide program development and maintenance with assurance of harmony between the interests of administration and the interests of clinical practice. Later in life I had the added privilege of learning from Milton Greenblatt, who wrote extensively on the theory and practice of psychiatric administration from a historical perspective. We collaborated on *Anatomy of Psychiatric Administration: The Organization in Health and Disease,* published in 1992.

Prior to the early 1980s the annual course offered at Albert Einstein College of Medicine by Seymour Kaplan, M.D., was the premiere if not the only educational program in the field of mental health administration; however, because sessions were scheduled every other week over an extended period of time, course attendance was practically limited to New

Yorkers. Unfortunately, Dr. Kaplan did not believe there would be sufficient interest in a nationally advertised course consolidated into several days. Fortunately, he agreed to be the keynote lecturer for my first annual (and consolidated) continuing education course on this topic, and, fortunately, the course was successful.

The nationally advertised, consolidated, annual course I introduced at Wright State University School of Medicine in Dayton, Ohio, primarily for psychiatrists interested in preparing for the APA-sponsored certification examination, evolved over the years to include representatives of all mental health disciplines as well as individuals trained exclusively in administration. It is noteworthy that, as the years passed, the course enrollment included more and more clinicians without direct involvement in administration. These participants expressed a strong need to know about the workings of mental health care delivery systems because of their awareness of the organization's influences on their clinical effectiveness and vice versa.

Awareness of another dynamic force—managed care—began modifying interest in the historical, theoretical, and heretofore practical administrative perspectives typically offered in courses. While the number of clinicians who participated in my course increased, so did the number of managed care companies influencing their practices and, perhaps, their availability for courses of this kind. Enrollment, affected by other factors as well, began to decline.

October 1996 marked the fifteenth and final annual continuing medical education course on administration of mental health services under my supervision. Throughout its history the course provided education for over a thousand participants, whose feedback enriched the course overall and especially the presentations by course faculty, most of whom returned from year to year. Not only are all the authors of this *Guide* involved in education on an ongoing basis; almost all served as faculty members for my course "New Dimensions in Mental Health Administration" sometime in its history. The content and delivery of information contained in this *Guide,* therefore, has been field-tested on the basis of the authors' interactions with discriminating audiences.

As evidenced by the wide range of involvement in mental health administration among course attendees—from full-time clinicians with curiosity about administration to clinicians serving as full-time executives to executives without clinical training—the information contained in this *Guide* is desirable if not essential for all professionals participating in mental health care delivery systems. Because most mental health care delivery these days is organization based, a practical understanding of the forces contributing to organization effectiveness is in the best interest of all service providers—and, ultimately, in the best interest of consumers. As stated previously, administration and service delivery are dynamically inseparable. This *Guide,* therefore, addresses issues germane to both "exclusively clinical" and "exclusively administrative" practices as well as the spectrum of role combinations in between.

As described by Ray Patterson in his chapter, "Review Mechanisms and Regulatory Agencies," the modern history of administration in psychiatry began in 1844 with the founding of the first medical specialty organization, the Association of Medical Superintendents of American Institutions for the Insane, which eventually became the American Psychiatric Association. In 1953 the APA established a Committee on Certification of Mental Hospital Administrators. In 1981 the committee was renamed the APA Committee on Administrative Psychiatry, and in 1997 it became the APA Committee on Psychiatric Administration and Management.

The course from which the chapters in this *Guide* originated was organized in accordance with the components of the certification examination conducted by the APA Committee on Psychiatric Administration and Management: administrative theory and human resources, psychiatric care management, fiscal management, and law and ethics. Information on this certification examination is available, by the way, through the Office of Education, American Psychiatric Association, 1400 K Street, NW, Washington, DC 20005.

Many professional associations stress the importance of expertise in mental health administration. The membership of the American Association of Psychiatric Administrators is limited to psychiatrists, while the membership of the American College of Mental Health Administration includes all mental health professionals. The Association of Mental Health Administrators, which is also multidisciplinary, offers a credentialing examination. The American College of Physician Executives is a rapidly expanding organization that offers educational programs and a credentialing examination to physicians in all specialties. The International Society for the Psychoanalytic Study of Organizations presents professional development workshops and annual symposia. Likewise, the Academy of Organizational and Occupational Psychiatry, founded in 1990, conducts annual educational programs. The American Psychiatric Association, the American Psychological Association, the National Association of Social Workers, and the American Psychiatric Nurses Association all sponsor presentations on administrative issues.

The chapters in this *Guide* provide information on the fundamental concepts and principles involved in the delivery of mental health services. It is important to note that its authors are not exclusively involved in education. Each also practices in the area of his or her expertise. The *Guide* is intended to educate readers on a practical level. It is a primer, not a textbook. A glossary is included for easy reference to definitions. The rationale for the order of chapters is based on external versus internal orientation from an organizational perspective. The beginning chapters address concepts and factors mostly external to the organization, and the final chapters describe activities mostly generated from inside the organization, although these activities are frequently carried out, in part, in response to influences of an external nature. Outcome studies, for example, are initiated and carried out internally, yet external (review and regulatory agency) expectations play a role in the process.

One major benefit of having served as the editor for the production of this *Guide* is the opportunity to revisit my former working relationships with its authors. I've known most for many years—Ric Reichard for twenty-five or more. Although the durations of my associations with the authors vary, my admiration of their respective talents does not. I am deeply indebted to all the authors for their willingness to share their wisdom in this publication, which provides readers with a distillation of the content of the long-lived course in which they taught. For me the *Guide* provides durable evidence of closure to a long-term commitment that embodied considerable meaning from both personal and professional points of view.

Glimpses of the authors' personalities and accomplishments can be obtained by reading between the lines. The benefits derived from Ken Gaver's expertise in mental health care administration are legion. His many achievements as an executive in both the public and private sectors and his leadership of the professional associations representing these interests have far-reaching ramifications. Ric Reichard has been enjoying a remarkably successful career as a consultant to health care systems and organizations and as an educator at American University. Marty Martin's knowledge of human resources dazzles everyone, and the many participants in my annual courses were no exception. I'm privileged to be instrumental in publishing "Patterson's Top-Ten Considerations for Preparation" for review by regulatory agencies. Ray's experience as a surveyor for the Joint Commission on Accreditation of Healthcare Organizations (JCAHO) has been invaluable to those interested in learning about review mechanisms and regulatory agencies.

Charles Scott, a forensic child and adolescent psychiatrist now at the University of California, Davis Campus, and author of the chapter "Mental Health Law," has proven repeatedly that wisdom is not limited to those in the zenith of their careers. The students, house officers, and faculty at Wright State University School of Medicine have been extremely fortunate to be able to count on Marshall Kapp and Doug Mossman for their unique combined perspectives—legal, public health, and medical—on health care issues, and Tonette Krousel-Wood has a similar following at Tulane University School of Medicine among those interested in public health. She serves as an admirable role model for combined MD/MPH degree candidates at Tulane.

Early in the history of my annual course on the administration of mental health care services, Dennis Staton helped identify and then filled a need for education on the national aspects of psychiatric care finance. Being a member of the course faculty from way back, Dennis began his career as a peripatetic expert in this field with clippings from the *Wall Street Journal.* Ray Newman's presentation of the basics of budgeting and hospital finance is so compelling it inspires interest in this subject even among dyed-in-the-wool clinicians. Likewise, Gordon Whyte's expertise in marketing mental health care has convinced course participants of the importance of applying these principles to their organizations.

In the course of my years of interest in the literature on administration of mental health care services I've discovered several gaps. Some of my attempts to develop or reinforce the literature in these areas seem to complement the information provided in this *Guide.* As a *lagniappe*—a Louisiana term for a little something extra—I've taken the liberty to list several review articles that might be of interest as supplementary reading. The topics include: the importance of cultural sensitivity to administration of mental health care services (Rodenhauser 1994); a psychodynamic perspective on organizational life, including regression (Rodenhauser 1993); the dynamics of the team approach to treatment (Rodenhauser 1996); the dynamically informed choice of a new leader (Rodenhauser and Senior 1995); and perceptions of the benefits and meaning of APA certification in administrative psychiatry (Rodenhauser, Hatchette, and Arce 1995).

The *Guide* in your hands is priority reading, however. I'm confident that the information contained herein will be of inestimable value in striving to improve the delivery of mental health care services in your organization.

REFERENCES

Rodenhauser, P. 1993. Regression as a cardinal factor in organizational destabilization. *Administration and Policy in Mental Health* 20:153–64.

Rodenhauser, P. 1994. Cultural barriers to mental health care delivery in Alaska. *Journal of Mental Health Administration* 21:60–70.

Rodenhauser, P. 1996. Psychiatrists as treatment team leaders: Pitfalls and rewards. *Psychiatric Quarterly* 67:11–31.

Rodenhauser, P., R. K. Hatchette, and A. A. Arce. 1995. A survey of psychiatrists with APA certification in administrative psychiatry. *Psychiatric Services* 46:1278–83.

Rodenhauser, P., and N. Senior. 1995. The dynamically informed choice of a new leader. *Administration and Policy in Mental Health* 23:3–15.

Contents

Chapter 1
The National Health Care Economic Context of Psychiatric Practice
R. Dennis Staton, Ph.D., M.D. 1

Chapter 2
Mental Health Care Delivery Systems
Kenneth Gaver, M.D. 31

Chapter 3
Marketing Mental Health Services
E. Gordon Whyte, Ph.D., and William F. Martin, Psy.D., M.P.H., M.A. 53

Chapter 4
Review Mechanisms and Regulatory Agencies
Raymond F. Patterson, M.D. 76

Chapter 5
Mental Health Law
Charles L. Scott, M.D. 101

Chapter 6
Documentation for Health Care Administrators
Marshall B. Kapp, J.D., M.P.H., and Douglas Mossman, M.D. 128

Chapter 7
Financial Management
Ray G. Newman, Ph.D. 148

Chapter 8
Managing Organization Behavior
Birge D. Reichard, Ph.D. 179

Chapter 9
Human Resources in Mental Health Care Organizations
William F. Martin, Psy.D., M.P.H., M.A. 201

Chapter 10
Outcomes Assessment and Performance Improvement: Measurements and Methodologies That Matter in Mental Health Care
Marie A. Krousel-Wood, M.D., M.S.P.H. 233

About the Authors 255

Index 259

CHAPTER 1

The National Health Care Economic Context of Psychiatric Practice

R. Dennis Staton, Ph.D., M.D.

The structure of health care insurance and delivery in the United States has been radically transformed during the last two decades of this century. The impact of this transformation upon consumer access, upon the treatments provided, and upon the administration of health care services has been enormous and problematic (Kassirer 1998). This impact has been especially difficult for psychiatric patients, practitioners, and administrators. The very nature of psychiatric practice, as it existed for the three decades prior to the late 1980s, has been (and continues to be) radically altered by powerful forces external to psychiatry (Staton 1989). Although this alteration has been facilitated by scientific and technologic discoveries, it has been driven primarily by nonmedical, societal factors. As a consequence, general medical and psychiatric administration have been made enormously more complex, difficult, and risky.

The goal of this chapter is to identify general principles and corollaries of these principles that can be used to clarify why health care insurance and delivery in the United States has changed, and will continue to change, so radically. The purpose for doing so is to facilitate the exercise of informed, realistic, and adaptive decision-making by psychiatric administrators and practitioners.

General Principles

Principle 1: Health care costs more than most payers can afford, or are willing, to pay.

Corollary: Most payers for health care will continue to constrain costs, or will attempt to avoid paying for health care altogether.

Employers

Employers pay approximately 24 percent of total U.S. health care expenditures, more than $230 billion in 1994 (Bodenheimer and Sullivan 1998b). In 1996 $1,200 of every General Motors' (GM) vehicle manufactured in the United States, more than twice the cost of the steel, represented the cost of GM's health benefits. GM's total health care expenditures in that year were $4.8 billion (Iglehart 1997). The high cost of health care has prompted most employers to abandon, as much as possible, responsibility for providing health insurance. They intend to pay the lowest practicable amount for the smallest number of employees that still permits them to recruit or retain necessary workers, who demand this benefit.

In industry after industry throughout the 1990s U.S. companies engaged in major restructuring to reduce costs and increase profits. This downsizing included significant reductions in health benefits. In 1990, 61 percent of the U.S. population was covered by employer-sponsored health insurance. Just four years later, in 1994, this percentage had fallen below 57 percent. Steady decline in employer-sponsored health insurance is expected to continue, though more slowly (Larkin 1996).

Employers have significantly increased required health benefit cost-sharing by insured employees (demand-side cost sharing) (Larkin 1996; Smith 1997; AFL-CIO 1998). The average premium paid by employees for individual coverage increased 284 percent between 1989 and 1996 (vs. total premium cost growth of 79 percent). The average premium paid by employees for family coverage increased 146 percent between 1989 and 1996 (vs. 111 percent for total cost growth during this period). The Lewin Group estimated that employee-paid premium expenditures could double between 1996 and 2002 (AFL-CIO 1998). Total premium costs—employers' plus employees' shares—are now less worrisome for employers, since they shift cost increases to their employees. Many low-income employees, even though they have access to employer-sponsored health insurance, cannot afford the required premium contributions and are forced to surrender their insurance coverage. This lowers organization health benefit expenditures even further. The American tradition of employers assuming primary responsibility for the cost of their employees' health insurance is rapidly being abandoned.

Medicare

There are approximately 38 million Medicare beneficiaries. This number will grow steadily until approximately the year 2011, when the large "baby boom" generation begins to retire and markedly increases both the number of beneficiaries and Medicare costs. The Medicare program pays 20 percent of total U.S. health care expenditures. Total Medicare costs for fiscal year (FY) 1998 are estimated to have been $208.6 billion, 12.3 percent of the total U.S. FY 1998 federal budget outlay. Medicare total cost is estimated to rise to $295.1 billion, 14.7 percent of the total, in FY 2002. The U.S. Office of Management and Budget (OMB) estimates that Medicare costs will grow at an average annual rate of 9 percent during the period FY 1996–2002, significantly outpacing general inflation (Analytical Perspectives 1998). By approximately the year 2011 the magnitude and the rate of growth of Medicare costs will not be sustainable by payroll tax revenues: "Medicare as we know it is unsustainable" (Gramm et al. 1998a). An alternative financing system must be developed that requires each generation to pay for its own retirement health care (Gramm et al. 1998b). Most important, **Medicare costs will have to be constrained much more aggressively.**

Medicaid

There are approximately thirty million low-income individuals enrolled in state Medicaid programs. Nationwide, these programs pay 14 percent of total U.S. health care expenditures.

During the 1980s and early 1990s Medicaid expenditures imposed huge burdens on state governments, even though the federal government pays, on average, 57 percent (and states only 43 percent) of total costs (Samuelson 1996). The average annual growth in Medicaid costs was 12.5 percent between 1980 and 1993 (Levit et al. 1995; Busch 1997). By 1994 Medicaid costs constituted 19 percent of state budgets (Samuelson 1996).

Aggressive cost-reduction actions by state governments during the early and mid-1990s markedly lowered the high rates of Medicaid cost inflation. Nonetheless, OMB estimates that federal Medicaid expenses will grow at an average annual rate of 7 percent during the period FY 1996–2002, again (like Medicare costs) significantly outpacing general inflation. Total federal expenses for Medicaid in FY 1998 are estimated to have been $104.5 billion, 6.2 percent of the total FY 1998 federal budget outlay. Federal Medicaid costs are projected to rise to $139.2 billion, 7.0 percent of the total, in FY 2002 (Analytical Perspectives 1998).

Mental Health Costs

Between 55 and 60 percent of total spending for mental health and substance abuse treatment in the United States, which was approximately $90 billion in 1998 (extrapolated from McKusick et al. 1998), is paid by the public sector: federal, state, and local governments (AHA 1997; McKusick et al. 1998). Medicaid and other state and local government programs pay for nearly 40 percent of the total; Medicare and other (non-Medicaid) federal programs pay for 17 percent (McKusick et al. 1998). Approximately 90 percent of total expenditures is consumed by the 15 percent of psychiatric patients with severe mental illness (AHA 1997).

The public sector share of total mental health and substance abuse treatment costs increased steadily between 1986 and 1996 (McKusick et al. 1998). By 1996 only 45 percent of admissions to private psychiatric units were covered by managed care contracts and commercial insurance; 48 percent of these admissions were covered by Medicaid, Medicare, or other government insurance (National Association 1997). Private insurance pays for only slightly more than 25 percent of total U.S. mental health and substance abuse treatment (McKusick et al. 1998). **Between 70–75 percent of total U.S. mental health and substance abuse treatment costs are funded by federal, state, and local governments and private out-of-pocket expenditures.**

The aggregate cost of treating mental illness and substance abuse in the United States ranks third in national spending for disease categories, behind spending for heart disease and for injury/trauma. In 1996 expenditures for mental health and substance abuse treatment services in the United States constituted 8.1 percent of total U.S. health care costs. The mental health and substance abuse treatment share was 9.0 percent in 1986. National spending for these services has steadily declined as a percentage of total U.S. health care spending. Approximately 84 percent of mental health and substance abuse treatment spending is for the treatment of mental illness; 16 percent is spent to treat alcohol and other drug abuse. Hospitals consume one-third of total U.S. mental health and substance abuse expenditures; psychiatrists, psychologists, counselors, and social workers consume only 17 percent of the total (McKusick et al. 1998).

During the years 1987–91 employer mental health benefit costs increased at annual rates between 21 percent and 27 percent, nearly double the 10 percent to 15 percent increases in total U.S. health care costs (WBGH 1996; AHA 1997). These mental health cost increases were primarily generated by inappropriate hospitalizations of adolescents with behavior problems and individuals with substance abuse diagnoses (AHA 1997). **Employers fear mental health benefit costs,** in part because of the subjective nature of psychiatric diagnoses and the professional disagreements about treatment planning. They view these benefits as discretionary and price-sensitive (higher out-of-pocket cost reduces demand from individual employees: demand for these benefits is elastic).

Individual Consumers

Individual consumers are very sensitive to even small differences in copay requirements or additional (out-of-pocket) costs associated with choosing a higher-cost health plan (Newhouse 1993; Busch 1997; Bodenheimer and Sullivan 1998a). When given a choice of provider coupled with copay responsibility, most individual consumers select lower-cost options. "Very small differences in price cause large movements of patients" (Ellwood 1997). Demand for mental health care is especially elastic (Newhouse 1993). Although consumers do want to have choice of physicians and to receive quality services, cost is the paramount concern.

Conclusion

All payers believe that their health care costs are too high. Their primary concern is direct cost, and they choose insurance plans with the lowest costs. Higher-cost plans, even if they are not-for-profit and provide better care, are infrequently selected (Stone 1998). As many authors have observed, the top three determinants of health care decision making are: (1) cost; (2) cost; and (3) cost. The only significant exception to this reality occurs among individuals who have important, specific treatment needs and choice (e.g., seriously ill Medicare beneficiaries). **All strategic planning by psychiatric administrators must emphasize cost of services as the most important determinant of organization survival.** Convenience and apparent quality of services are important, but much less so (Bodenheimer and Sullivan 1998b). Mental health costs are of particular concern to payers, for reasons noted in the preceding two sections.

Principle 2: The structure of health insurance and delivery in the United States has become predominantly corporate and for-profit.

Corollary: Managers of health care insurance organizations are primarily profit-oriented.

Corporatization of Health Care Delivery

Marmor (1998:552) describes Americans in the 1990s as "living in the twilight of the earlier Golden Age (of Medicine)." This earlier age was "golden" for physicians and their patients, but not for the payers of health care. The subsequent transformation of the U.S. health care system, in both organization form and the locus of medical authority (Marmor

1998), was directed at: (1) reducing rates of growth in the cost of health care; and (2) obtaining profits. The largest industry in the nation became entrepreneurial, corporate, for-profit, shareholder-owned (Kuttner 1998a). "For-profit . . . health plans (have expanded) at a much greater rate than their not-for-profit competitors" (Schroeder 1996). Marmor aptly identifies these new corporate forms as "health finance organizations" not managed care organizations (Marmor 1998:562), because they typically display little evidence of caring about patients. "Managed care in practice has mostly meant cutting back on payment levels, medical choices, and covered services . . . It has been largely the 'managing' of costs, not the micromanaging of care" (Marmor 1998:562; see also Hacker 1997b). Retrospective, cost-based, fee-for-service reimbursement has been replaced by prospective (including capitation) payment. Providers now have a reversed (and perverse) incentive: **providing fewer medical services produces more profit.** Most managed care insurers are commercial businesses seeking profits in the trillion dollar a year U.S. health care industry, with fiduciary responsibilities to optimize profitability for the benefit of shareholders.

Managed care insurer organizations have depended on investors and borrowed capital to fuel their astonishing growth. The early, spectacular cost savings, produced by demanding large discounts from hospitals and physicians, stimulated capital investment. By the fourth quarter of 1996, however, the average operating profit margin of publicly traded, managed care corporations had evaporated to –1.1 percent (Hilzenrath 1997), because many had bought market share by underpricing their insurance (Iglehart 1997), and because significant additional cost reductions are difficult to achieve. Provider resistance to further discounting has hardened. The provider-squeezing strategy has reached the point of diminishing (or vanishing) returns. The cost impact of expensive technologic innovations is difficult to contain. Premium price increases brought the average profit margin of managed care corporations to +0.9 percent in the first quarter of 1997; prices are expected to continue increasing, by 5 percent to 8 percent a year (Hilzenrath 1997). Premium inflation, the shrinking profit margins, the high risk, and the 1998 stock market contractions are likely to reduce managed care insurers' ability to attract capital.

Effect of Corporatization

The new corporate, for-profit managed care insurers markedly constrain health care expenditures, primarily by sharply reducing access to (and utilization of) hospital beds and medical specialists (Stone 1998). The earlier retrospective, cost-based, fee-for-service U.S. health care system, with its incentive to provide more and more care, had produced significant excess capacity. Between 1984 and 1995, the new market forces closed nearly 600 hospitals and eliminated 260,000 hospital beds (Schroeder 1996) and markedly restricted access to specialist services. Although hospitals still consume approximately 32 percent, more than $350 billion per year, of total U.S. health care expenditures, they have been displaced from the centers of health care delivery. The number of empty beds in surviving hospitals increases every year, down to an occupancy rate of 60 percent in 1997. Hospital consolidations and closures will continue. In this respect, and others, the health care delivery industry is undergoing forced downsizing comparable to that of American industry in general in the 1990s.

Corporate, for-profit, managed care organizations offer health insurance at lower annual costs than did traditional not-for-profit plans or traditional indemnity insurers. At the same time, they provide appreciably less health care per premium dollar. They spend, on average, only 65–85 percent of each premium dollar for health care (which they identify as their "medical-loss ratio") (Herzlinger 1997; Kuttner 1998a). Traditional indemnity insurers and major not-for-profit plans spend 90 percent or more of every premium dollar for health care; for example, considerably less for administrative and marketing expenses and profits (Herzlinger 1997; Kuttner, 1998a; 1998b). For-profit managed care insurers do lower the overall cost of health care, but because they spend large amounts on administration, advertising, and stockholders' profits (Kassirer 1998), they provide substantially less care than did traditional insurers. They also are much less willing to pay for uncompensated and discounted care (Schroeder 1996; Smith 1997; Thorpe 1997).

Quality of Corporate Care

Does forced reduction of resources allocated for health care—and the consequent provision of less care—result in frequent provision of inadequate care? Numerous published reports of individual instances of substandard care and a small number of research studies confirm that this is the case (Hacker 1997b; Ware 1996). Managed care reviewers often, if not generally, search for justification to not authorize requested treatments (because they are not indicated, nonstandard, experimental, or whatever) (Herzlinger 1997). Even though HMOs have been shown to deliver certain medical services with no decrement, or even with some improvement, in quality (e.g., preventive evaluations and treatments in relatively healthy populations of patients), there is a considerable body of evidence that frequently they provide inadequate care for certain medical conditions and perhaps for most major psychiatric illness (Herzlinger 1997; Chang et al. 1998).

Many authors assume that the provision of less care is synonymous with providing care of unacceptable quality (Kassirer 1998; Stone 1998). This premise is difficult to document. The question, "What is appropriate care?" is presently unanswerable; suggested answers are significantly arbitrary (Naylor 1998). The benefits of medical or psychiatric treatments can range from prevention of serious harm to limited improvements in functional status. How much benefit does society (employers, governments, individual payers, and voters) wish to insure? To pay for? These are not questions of quality per se, unless high quality is defined as maximum achievable benefit (at any cost). Even if the criteria used to answer this question were scientific, not economic, "there are many gray areas of clinical practice in which evidence about benefits is incomplete or conflicting" (Naylor 1998:1920, 1995). This observation is particularly true with respect to the practice of psychiatry.

Nonetheless, Kassirer is correct in worrying that "physicians will be under great pressure to provide even less than minimally accepted care" (Kassirer 1998:398; see also Kassirer 1995; 1997; Latham 1996). He is also correct in observing that a corollary of our present inability to define and monitor quality is a corresponding inability to monitor and document unacceptable undertreatment. To date, managed care insurers have been relatively free to ignore quality as a serious issue, because their misleading marketing promises of better, more comprehensive, and preventive care cannot (yet) be convincingly refuted.

The Form of Managed Care

The central feature of corporate managed care development in the 1980s and 1990s has been the consolidation, in single organizations, of two previously separate roles: the role of insurance company/fiscal intermediary and the role of health care provider (Rettig 1997; Stone 1998). The major, traditional, indemnity health insurers became, wholly or in large part, managed care insurance corporations by contracting with and/or purchasing provider businesses, to form **integrated insurance-delivery systems** (Robinson 1994; Shortell et al. 1995; Stoeckle 1995; Struss and Halleland 1998). Network forms of managed care delivery (in contrast with staff- and group-model HMOs) are most popular with patients and have garnered a majority share of the managed care market, because they permit enrollees a greater choice of providers (Herzlinger 1997). Physician members of this form of managed care organization, however, have considerably less influence over treatment intrusions by organization administrations (Kuttner 1998a).

In many U.S. markets the buyer monopoly for physician services is controlled by small numbers of large (and growing), vertically integrated managed care insurers. Although the vertically integrated structure of these organizations appears to presage the future of health care delivery in the United States, ownership of hospitals and other subsidiary business components (including physician groups) creates financial liability, not economic advantage. Economically, it is more sensible to rent these resources when they are needed. Herzlinger emphasizes that vertical integration (ownership of multiple vertical business components) "confers benefits only in special circumstances" (Herzlinger 1997:147), that is, when there is need to secure necessary resources that are in short supply. Few health care delivery resources are in short supply. Vertically integrated organizations are very difficult to manage cost-effectively, in part because the component subsidiaries are protected from external competition; they become in-house, inefficient (more expensive) suppliers of services. Moreover, vertically integrated, for-profit organizations have an inherent tendency to avoid price competition with competitors (Herzlinger 1997): reducing prices reduces profitability and lowers returns for shareholders. Therefore, our current large, vertically integrated health care organizations are unlikely, in the long run, to achieve the cost efficiencies and lower prices they have promised to employer and governmental payers (Relman 1998).

If payers and networks of physician and hospital providers (provider-sponsored organizations, PSOs) were able to contract directly with each other, they could eliminate the serious disadvantages (financial waste, loss of medical authority) that are associated with the intermediary function of the for-profit managed care insurers. For this alternative to become viable, payer coalitions and PSOs would have to grow appreciably in numbers and strength (Bodenheimer and Sullivan 1998b). PSOs would also have to develop capital financing, management skill, and the capacity to successfully assume the financial risk associated with managing the health care of defined populations (Ginzberg and Ostow 1997). Although direct payer-provider contracting is not (yet) viable in most markets (Ginzberg and Ostow 1997; Bodenheimer and Sullivan 1998a; 1998b), health care providers increasingly are consolidating into larger groups with more bargaining power (Foster Higgins 1997). PSOs that are able to develop the requisite strength and administrative expertise—and that remain not-for-profit and genuinely physician-managed—will have considerable potential to reestablish physician influence and bargaining power in the health care marketplace and, at the same time, to markedly reduce the billions of U.S. health care dollars now being wasted on unnecessary corporate administrative, marketing, and profit-margin expenses.

Employer and governmental payers and large insurers frequently use national, for-profit mental health and substance abuse managed care corporations (managed behavioral health care vendors) to separately manage and pay for all of their mental health and substance abuse treatment care (behavioral health carve-outs) (Ettner and Notman 1997; Hodgkin et al. 1997). Nearly 150 million Americans are insured for mental health and substance abuse services through managed behavioral health care carve-outs (Managed Care 1998). For state government payers, this process of **privatization,** "contracting with private sector providers for services previously supplied by the public sector" (Libby 1997), constitutes a major transformation of mental health and substance abuse treatment financing.

The three largest managed behavioral health care corporations cover 90 million individuals; the ten largest companies cover 80 percent of all mental health and substance abuse treatment carve-out enrollees (Managed Care 1998). Rapidly evolving horizontal and vertical consolidation within the managed behavioral health care industry is producing fewer, larger companies competing for private and public, managed mental health and substance abuse treatment contracts (Emery et al. 1998). Large managed behavioral health care corporations are better able, than smaller organizations, to operate efficiently and assume risk in this early period of market restructuring, which increases their likelihood of short-term survival and achievement of oligopolistic management of the nation's $90 billion mental health system (McKusick et al. 1998). To the extent that state mental health dollars become integrated with social service monies (e.g., case management, child protection, juvenile justice, special education, etc.) (Emery et al. 1998), the potential profit for managed behavioral health care vendors is even greater.

Health maintenance organizations (HMOs) have the option of providing their own internal mental health services. To do so requires a sufficiently large number of covered lives, logistical convenience for patients, and very tight management of cost efficiency. HMOs with internal provision can still contract out for specific, specialized psychiatric services (specialized niche contracts) (Hodgkin et al. 1997).

Not-for-Profit Delivery Systems

Not-for-profit delivery systems must aggressively and successfully compete with large for-profit corporations for market share, that is, they must offer payers comparably low prices (as well as acceptable quality) for their medical services. In order to do so, they must employ very similar marketing and financial management strategies. The current market-driven incentive is for all provider organizations, for-profit and not-for-profit, to minimize resources (including clinician time) expended for treatment.

The Health Care Free Market

Since mid-1994, when the Clinton administration's proposed Health Security bill was stalemated in Congress (Hacker 1997a; Marmor 1998), "free market" capitalism has emerged as the de facto U.S. national health policy (Schroeder 1996), directed primarily at controlling runaway cost inflation, but also seeking attractive profits, essentially unregulated by governmental oversight (Kassirer 1997). "Politicians of both parties promote managed care as the best way to control Medicare and Medicaid costs" (Schroeder 1996). Indeed, management of care has been significantly successful in reducing cost inflation. At the same time, however, the new market economy, which does not provide goods for free, has undermined the clinical revenue source of funding for this country's medical infrastructure (medical education, clinical research, some aspects of public health) and the safety nets for indigent care (Schroeder 1996). The competitive free market will not voluntarily subsidize, in significant degree, these social needs. Competitive advantage is gained by not incurring these costs (Ginzberg and Ostow 1997). Managed health care is a free market for corporate for-profit entrepreneurs, not for American health care consumers.

Hacker (1997b) concludes that the current Madison Avenue rhetoric about a free market in the health care industry cannot come to fruition because this market does not function as a normal consumer market. "In the real world of health care finance . . . markets are necessarily supported and policed by government" (Hacker 1997b:1447). Stone (1998), paraphrasing Lester Thurow of the Massachusetts Institute of Technology, emphasizes the additional, important point that "free markets . . . cannot solve (the) ethical problems of equitable distribution" of health care in the U.S. "Government regulation will be needed to protect the public interest" (Relman 1998). Managed care's for-profit domination of U.S. health care will harm many patients. Governments must "set the balance points" between cost reduction/profit-taking and consumer protection (Schroeder 1996; Ginzberg and Ostow 1997).

Schroeder identifies six national health policy dilemmas which must be solved: (1) Should everyone have the right to basic health care? (2) To what extent should the healthy subsidize the sick or the wealthy subsidize the poor? (3) What is government's role in health care? (4) Is medicine merely a business like any other? (5) Should there be limits on the profits obtained from providing health care services? and (6) How do we best invest in medicine's future—in research and training? (1996:20). These problems must be solved by federal and state governments. The for-profit health care free market cannot, and should not be allowed to, provide de facto solutions.

The Decline of Funding for Charity Care

The number of Americans covered by employer-sponsored health insurance is steadily declining. "A permanent contraction in the private insurance market is under way" (Smith 1997:1000), which represents a "radical restructuring of health care financing" in the United States (Larkin 1996:2). At the same time, the number of individuals eligible for Medicaid insurance is tightly constrained and is declining for some populations (Smith 1997). As a consequence, the numbers of uninsured and underinsured Americans are steadily rising (Schroeder 1996; AHA 1997; Ginzberg and Ostow 1997; Smith 1997)—more than 44 million people were uninsured in 1997 (Schroeder 1997).

Disadvantaged Americans traditionally received charity care from not-for-profit hospitals, which was funded by cross-subsidies taken from inflated charges to private payers and from Medicare profits. As payments for the hospital treatment of private and Medicare patients have been reduced by managed care and the Health Care Financing Administration (HCFA), however, and as the number of employer-insured individuals has declined, most of the financial margins that not-for-profit hospitals once used to subsidize charity care have been eliminated. As a consequence, the amount of uncompensated care being provided is declining (Smith 1997), while the need for *more* uncompensated care is increasing (Larkin 1996). Hospitals can attempt to cope with this situation by shifting costs to those employers who still provide health benefits, but this raises these employers' costs and undermines their willingness to continue providing health benefits. As a result of these factors, the nation "is on the brink of a major collision" between the increasing need for uncompensated care and the decreasing financial capacity of traditional safety-net providers to deliver this care (Smith 1997:1001).

Since indigent care is insufficiently subsidized in the corporate managed care marketplace, insurance for uninsured and underinsured individuals must be subsidized or provided *by governments.* Efforts to provide this protection, even if very basic, must be genuine and tangible—not illusory, such as vouchers or tax credits (Smith 1997). Although U.S. society tolerates considerable covert (implicit) rationing of the health care services made available to its poor (Schroeder 1996), it will not tolerate their explicit exclusion from care. "Governments will be forced to act" (Ginzberg and Ostow 1997:1020). The national cost of universal coverage would amount to only $20 billion a year (2 percent of total U.S. health care expenditures) (Schroeder 1996).

Who Administers?

In this environment of nearly unrestrained for-profit, entrepreneurial, corporate competition, senior and mid-level administrators need financial, marketing, production line, and risk-management expertise. Only a small number of physicians is likely to develop this necessary level of corporate business expertise. Medical or psychiatric training is optional. Accordingly, nearly all physicians will function as expendable "employees at will," whether they are salaried or reimbursed for services provided.

Principle 3: Payers for health care (employers, governments, and managed care insurers) have enormous power to dictate (changes in) what specific medical treatments will be reimbursed, how many of these treatments will be permitted (reimbursed), and how much will be paid for each treatment.

Corollary: Given Principle 1 and its corollary, most payers for health care will continue to demand and obtain stringent cost containment from health care providers.

Employers

Bodenheimer and Sullivan (1998a; 1998b) review the history of the pivotal role that large American corporations, using their enormous purchasing power, played in aggressively implementing new health insurance-purchasing strategies in the 1980s and 1990s, in order to reduce their escalating insurance costs. The most important of these strategies was the forced channeling of employees into managed care plans. In 1987, 92 percent of medium-sized and large employers utilized traditional fee-for-service indemnity insurance as their predominant method of paying for health care (Hay Group 1998). By 1997, 30 percent of insured employees were enrolled in traditional health maintenance organizations (HMOs), 35 percent in preferred provider organizations (PPOs), 20 percent in point-of-service (POS) plans, and only 15 percent in indemnity insurance plans (Foster Higgins 1998). Most employers now require managed care enrollment, with each employee receiving a fixed-dollar contribution per annum, which is either implicit or explicit. Many employers assign their employees to a single provider plan, with no choice, while others offer the option of selecting a higher-cost plan or out-of-plan physicians, provided that the employees pay all additional costs incurred (Bodenheimer and Sullivan 1998a; Kuttner 1998b). The average cost per active employee for HMO coverage, in 1997, was 10 percent less than the cost of managed indemnity insurance; it was 6 percent less for PPO coverage, but only 1 percent less for POS coverage (open-access HMOs) (Foster Higgins 1998).

Medium-sized and large private employers' costs for health insurance increased very little, or actually declined, between 1988 and 1997 (Foster Higgins 1997; Hay Group 1998). Employers attribute this impressive moderation of their health benefit cost increases primarily to their enrollment of employees in managed care plans, especially HMOs (Foster Higgins 1997). During the period 1993–96 the cumulative cost growth was only 3 percent for employer HMO premiums and 8 percent for PPO premiums, but 29 percent for indemnity plan expenses (Foster Higgins 1997). In reality much of the employer health cost moderation of the early 1990s had little to do with the operations of managed care (Ginsberg and Pickreign 1996). Cost shifting to employees and the reduction in the proportion of employees participating in employer-sponsored health insurance were major contributors to the slowed growth of employer costs.

The U.S. Department of Labor (Office of the Chief Economist 1996) attributes this health insurance cost reduction to: declining medical inflation (from nearly 10 percent in 1990 down to slightly over 5 percent in 1995 [Schroeder 1996]), expanded reliance upon managed care provision of health benefits (from approximately 25 percent enrollment in 1989 to 85 percent in 1997 [Foster Higgins 1998]), expanding numbers of employees who are required to share increasing percentages of the costs of employer-sponsored health insurance, and declining numbers of full-time workers (and retirees) participating in employer-sponsored health insurance (this primarily derives from significant reduction in the number of employees who can afford required cost sharing, but also includes a significant reduction in the number of employees and retirees offered employer-sponsored health benefits).

Conversion of employers' health benefits from traditional, high cost, fee-for-service, indemnity insurance to managed care insurance produced a relatively immediate, one-time cost reduction of 10 percent to 15 percent (Ginzberg and Ostow 1997). Once employees are enrolled in some form of managed care plan, however, additional cost savings are difficult to generate. The practice patterns of physicians and hospitals and the health care choices of enrollees cannot be constricted very much more. Access to medical technological innovation, a significant contributor to cost inflation (Rettig 1994; Ginzberg and Ostow 1997; Rettig 1997), but also a "primary guarantor of quality in U.S. health care" (Rettig 1997:3), is difficult to restrict without causing adverse publicity and increased exposure to malpractice litigation. In spite of aggressive management of the costs of care, we can anticipate relentless increase in both employer and national health care costs, in the absence of explicit rationing, and relentless pressure from payers to constrain these cost increases.

Employers expect the rate of growth of their health benefit premiums to increase in coming years, because: (1) most insured employees are now enrolled in managed care health plans; and (2) providers are consolidating to gain bargaining power with managed care insurers (Foster Higgins 1997). In addition, Medicare payment reductions will increase cost shifting to private payers. Employer pressure to constrain health care inflation and expenditures will therefore have to continue (Bodenheimer and Sullivan 1998b). Large employers and employer coalitions will use their extraordinary bargaining power to severely constrain the amounts of their annual fixed contributions per employee (Bodenheimer and Sullivan 1998a) and their total health care expenditures.

Both small and large employers can increase their negotiating power with health care insurance or provider organizations by aligning themselves in regional, joint-purchasing coalitions (Bodenheimer and Sullivan 1998a). This permits collective negotiation of a single, low premium rate for health insurance for each member employer with each competing managed care plan, for an agreed-upon standard set of benefits (Bodenheimer and Sullivan 1998a). Provided that a coalition controls a significant segment of the available market (and provided that the insurer-provider market is competitive), insurers and providers must accommodate coalition demands for cost containment or risk losing significant market share and revenue.

Managed Care Insurers

Managed care insurers achieve their power to force provider concessions by first gaining significant market share. They then can successfully demand discounts and shift financial risk to physicians and hospitals through withholds, capitation payments, and threats of deselection. In regions of the United States that have high penetration of large managed care insurers, there are many physician and hospital sellers of services but only a small number of insurer buyers (Stone 1998). As a consequence, insurers are able to conduct "shadow buying" of physician and other health care services and "shadow pricing" of premium rates to employers: competitor insurers follow suit (Moran 1998). As a group, the insurers become monopoly purchasers of physician and other services. Most physicians and other providers have no choice but to accept take-it-or-leave-it contracts (Moran 1998), because there are no other buyers. They have little or no negotiating power for either the price of their services or the terms of their contracts (Moran 1998). **There is a buyer monopoly for physician services.**

Managed care insurers increasingly use methods of payment that transfer some or all of their financial risk to their providers. These risk-shifting methods of payment include capitation, case rates, and the use of withholds or bonuses tied to achievement of specific cost-containment goals (Pearson et al. 1998; Struss and Halleland 1998). Use of capitation payment, a prospectively determined, flat rate per covered person, is rapidly becoming the primary method of paying providers of health care in the United States (Gabel 1997; Kassirer 1998; Physician Payment Review Commission 1996a; 1996b). With this payment method, providers receive fixed revenues and share (or assume all of) the risk of financial losses. Accordingly, they have very strong incentives to provide less care and to avoid assuming responsibility for seriously ill (expensive) patients, in order to avoid losses and maximize profits (Ettner and Notman 1997). Case rate payment of a fixed fee per treated patient per year, regardless of severity of illness or intensity of treatment need, carries an even greater financial risk for providers, and therefore an even greater incentive to minimize the care provided. Significant conflict of interest is also created when payment involves the use of withholds or bonuses and the amounts to be earned are large. Risk of financial loss can be mitigated by stop-loss insurance and/or risk pooling arrangements (Pearson et al. 1998).

When insurers experience financial pressure and are unable to raise premium rates to a sufficient level, they must reduce the capitation rates they pay to their providers. Their physicians and other clinicians are told (again) that they are providing too much care or are being paid too much. After another round of reimbursement reductions is put in place, access to services will become even more difficult and consumer confidence in the care being provided will be lessened even further (Moran 1998).

Employer Mental Health Benefits

Between 1988 and 1997 the average annual cost of U.S. employers' mental health benefits declined from 6–9 percent to just over 3 percent of total employer health costs (Patterson 1993; AHA 1997; Hodgkin et al. 1997; Hay Group 1998). Cost reductions were significantly greater for enrollees of managed care plans than they were for enrollees of indemnity plans (AHA 1997).

Medium-sized and large U.S. businesses reduced their spending for mental health and substance abuse services by 54.1 percent during the period 1988–97. This decrease was seven times greater than the 7.4 percent reduction in general medical benefit costs that occurred during this period. Total corporate health care cost reduction was 10.2 percent, in constant dollars, between 1988 and 1997 (Hay Group 1998); one-quarter of this total came from the marked decrease in psychiatric expenditures. The National Association of Psychiatric Health Systems (NAPHS), in its 1997 Annual Survey Report news release, anticipated that ". . . the pressure to reduce (mental health) costs has not abated—and may in fact be escalating" (NAPHS 1997).

Parity

The American Psychiatric Association and the National Alliance for the Mentally Ill have lobbied strenuously for "parity" insurance coverage for mental illness. Although these efforts have met with considerable state and federal legislative success, including the Mental Health Parity Act of 1996, they are meaningless (Stone 1998) because in managed care insurance plans the amount of insurance for mental illness treatments does not guarantee access, especially to expensive treatments (e.g., hospitalization, longer lengths of stay, and long-term psychotherapy). The fact that treatments are covered is irrelevant if they can be accessed only through gatekeepers who are paid to deny access and are authorized to reject the medical necessity of requested treatments. Managed care plans do not deliver all of the services covered by their benefit packages (Hodgkin et al. 1997; Sturm 1997) and parity legislation alone will not solve this barrier to equitable access.

Medicare

The Balanced Budget Act of 1997 (BBA 97) mandated $116.3 billion in Medicare spending reductions during the five-year period FY 1998 through FY 2002. Two-thirds of these reductions comes from Medicare fee-for-service payments to hospitals and physicians; nearly one-fifth comes from prospective payments to Medicare HMOs (Iglehart 1998). Psychiatric hospitals and psychiatric units of general hospitals, exempt from Medicare's Prospective Payment System, received major reductions in payments. Congress required 56.5 percent of the total BBA 1997 cost reduction to come from the Medicare Program, even though this Program constituted only 12–13 percent of the federal budget: strong evidence of Congress' intent to constrain Medicare costs.

Congress is relying upon three primary strategies to reduce Medicare growth: (1) reducing fee-for-service payments to providers; (2) shifting more costs to Medicare beneficiaries; and (3) increasing the enrollment of Medicare beneficiaries in managed care (prospective, capitation payment) programs. Congress is also experimenting with the ill-conceived medical savings accounts proposal. Strategies 1 and 2 have obvious limitations. If fee-for-service payments are decreased excessively, providers will avoid Medicare recipients or be bankrupted if Medicare losses cannot be shifted to other payers. It is likely that the political power of Medicare beneficiaries will defeat any large proposed increases in cost sharing, including increases in deductible/copayment requirements, a significant increase in the age of eligibility (e.g., to age seventy), or benefit package reductions (Angell 1997).

Medicare HMOs (Angell 1997; Morgan et al. 1997) are paid, for each enrollee, regardless of health status, 95 percent of the average annual cost for Medicare fee-for-service beneficiaries in their region (Angell 1997). There is no risk adjustment. Because Medicare HMOs selectively enroll healthier Medicare recipients and their sicker patients selectively disenroll to obtain HMO-denied benefits from the fee-for-service sector, the Medicare managed care strategy actually pays its HMO providers appreciably more for patient care than it would if these enrollees were to receive fee-for-service care (Angell 1997; Ginzberg and Ostow 1997; Morgan et al. 1997; Smith 1997). Moreover, the adverse selection for the fee-for-service system increases the capitation rate paid to Medicare HMOs to treat relatively healthy enrollees. Although the Department of Health and Human Services has proposed reduction of its Medicare HMO capitation payment by 7 percent (Ginzberg and Ostow 1997), accurate risk adjustment technology is not available. The managed care strategy for Medicare cost reduction, including the new PSO direct-contract option, is unlikely to succeed. This is especially so, because Medicare beneficiaries are the only sizable population in the United States that retains free choice in health care, and they are unwilling to trade this freedom for cost savings. Only 11 percent of Medicare beneficiaries had been attracted to Medicare HMOs by 1997 (Angell 1997).

Medicare represents the main alternative to corporate, for-profit managed care: a single-payer, fee-for-service system with very low administrative costs and free choice of physicians, hospitals, and other providers. Though subject to abuse by fraudulent providers, it has been an extremely successful program (Angell 1997). We may be fortunate that our most medically vulnerable individuals have both political power and belief that the fee-for-service Medicare system (of "socialized medicine") offers them better care when they are seriously ill. The critical problem of Medicare costs will have to be solved by Congress itself, not by profit-driven medical capitalism. Explicit rationing will have to be addressed.

State Mental Health Agencies

State mental health agencies historically have served as regulators, payers, and providers of mental health care (Emery et al. 1998). They control approximately 80 percent of all public monies spent for services provided to severely mentally ill individuals (Lynch 1997). State efforts to reduce

Medicaid cost growth—by constraining eligibility, reducing access to or eliminating certain benefits, and reducing reimbursements—have been insufficient. Although some state governments continue to rely on these measures, most others are converting the financing of their Medicaid mental health care with HCFA waiver authorization from fee-for-service or grant programs to capitated, risk-based, carve-out contracts with private managed behavioral health care vendors (Busch 1997; Emery et al. 1998)—or to a lesser extent with state-based public providers. Managed behavioral health care bidders must be sufficiently large to manage the administrative, service-delivery, and risk-assumption requirements of state Medicaid contracts. With managed behavioral health care contracting, **the market sets capitation rates** through competitive bidding (Busch 1997).

State mental health systems have been transformed by this use of private, capitated managed behavioral health care. The managed behavioral health care vendors serve as fiscal and management intermediaries between state payers and the clinical providers. They select the provider network and control utilization. As a result, states are now accountable for publicly funded services delivered in the private sector, as well as being responsible for surviving publicly operated services (Emery et al. 1998).

States believe that the use of at-risk, capitated carve-outs: (1) reduces the cost of their mental health benefits; (2) shifts financial risk exposure and the costs of bearing risk; (3) provides the expertise needed for the management of mental health benefits; and (4) increases alternate service options, e.g., new community services needed to permit reduced use of hospitalization (Busch 1997; Hodgkin et al. 1997). The major problem for payers of managed behavioral health care contracts is that these vendors, in search of market share and profits, may reduce expenditures and quality of care below accepted standards, increasing accusations of malpractice (and litigation exposure) (Hodgkin et al. 1997). Risk of substandard care is especially high, because these public/private partnerships (National Association 1997; Emery et al. 1998) must absorb diminishing public funding—already seriously deficient—for general health care and psychiatric illness (compare the BBA 1997-mandated $7.2 billion in Medicaid spending reductions during the five-year period FY 1998 through FY 2002; and the 1997 federal restriction of the use of Medicaid Disproportionate Share monies to support state psychiatric hospitals) (Emery et al. 1998) and also produce profits for managed behavioral health care shareholders. States are paying private (and some public) organizations to manage the provision of public care and, at the same time, to solve the problem of diminishing public allocations for mental health care.

The use of a private managed behavioral health care vendor by the

State of Massachusetts paid on a capitated basis has been associated with substantial problems with: integration of mental health services; linkages with support services; excessively slow verification of the eligibility of potential recipients; denial of reimbursement or late payment for services that had been authorized and provided; and poor, confusing, delayed communications about frequent changes in the rules of operation (Beinecke and Lockhart 1998).

State and county governments can continue to provide many services internally, contracting with private-sector providers for expensive services such as day care, inpatient, and residential treatment. In order for private sector procurement to reduce costs, however, there must be a competitive market of specialized providers (Libby 1997).

Conclusion

Employer and government payers for health care insurance and their agents, the large managed care insurers, have achieved essentially absolute power to control health care practice in the United States. Although consumers have considerable potential power (through state legislatures and Congress), it is unlikely that they will effect, in the foreseeable future, anything other than marginal adjustments in the rules of operation of health plans, Medicare, and Medicaid (Marmor 1998; Kuttner 1998b). We live in a political climate hostile to federal planning (Relman 1998). Physicians and other clinicians will remain relatively powerless to shape macroeconomic aspects of health care delivery. Even though the structure and functioning of managed care insurers is problematic, more state and federal regulation is probable, and physician-hospital networks are gaining strength, these for-profit insurers appear likely to retain their positions of power (Kassirer 1997).

Principle 4: Reduction of payments for medical services (receiving fewer dollars per year per covered individual) forces providers to increase productivity and/or decrease costs (personnel, resource utilization, overhead) while continuing to deliver an acceptable level of care that minimizes risk of costly illness relapses or litigation.

Insurer Cost Reduction

Managed care insurers reduce treatment costs by: (1) reducing access to expensive diagnostic procedures; (2) reducing access to expensive treatments (i.e., hospitalization, specialist care, surgery); (3) constricting the frequency of certain treatments; and (4) decreasing reimbursements for diagnostic procedures and treatments. Gatekeepers (primary care physicians and nonphysician reviewers) severely restrict access to all expensive diagnostic procedures and treatments for which "medical necessity" is not unequivocal.

The number of psychiatric inpatient admissions per 1000 people declined by approximately 35 percent from 1991 through 1996. Average psychiatric inpatient lengths of stay declined from 17.0 days in 1991 to 8.5 days in 1996 (Hay Group 1998). Mental health providers are treating outpatients with fewer visits per year for substantially lower payments per treatment (National Association 1997; Goldman et al. 1998; Sturm and McCulloch 1998). Outpatient visits per patient per year declined from 23.5 in 1994, to 15.4 in 1995, to 8.7 in 1996 (National Association 1997). The average payment per outpatient encounter decreased by 7.0 percent between 1991 and 1996 after adjusting for inflation (Hay Group 1998).

Coping with Reduced Revenue

Providers of general medical and psychiatric services must deliver quality services with finite, limited resources. This task can be facilitated by optimizing early diagnosis of and intervention with illnesses and episodes of clinical worsening.

Providers must cope with reductions of treatment revenue by: (1) increasing the productivity per hour of a smaller number of clinician hours; (2) reducing clinicians' salary per hour; or (3) successfully opposing insurer cost reduction demands. To the extent that clinicians are limited in their capacity to increase the number of treatment episodes processed per hour, they must either accept lower salaries for standard work weeks or work additional hours in order to maintain level incomes. Physicians working under capitation contracts can increase their incomes by accepting responsibility for greater numbers of covered lives, spending less time with these patients, delegating care to nonphysician assistants, and expending fewer resources per patient (Stone 1998).

Increasing productivity per hour beyond a certain point, however, jeopardizes the integrity of medical and psychiatric practice. At this point in time, adequate practice of psychiatry depends in significant degree upon careful assessments of subjective symptoms reported by patients who are variably able to communicate this information efficiently. Moreover, many patient encounters involve complex comorbidity, diagnostic uncertainty, concern about safety, and/or treatment dilemmas. These situations cannot be assessed and treated adequately during very brief clinical encounters. There clearly are limits to the number of outpatient visits that can be processed with acceptable quality per hour by a single clinician. To the extent that a number of clinical assistants could simultaneously elicit required information from different patients and provide necessary physician assistance and patient education, individual psychiatrists might successfully examine (and generate revenue from) many more patients per hour. This practice style, however, greatly increases the incidence of clinical mistakes. Managed care then becomes a process of managing the risk of expensive physician errors.

Psychiatric hospitals must now provide a range of alternative treatment services; admissions increasingly are to services other than inpatient hospitalization. Partial hospitalizations are increasing but with fewer average visits (National Association 1997). Managed care denials have dismantled the infrastructure of long-term psychiatric care, that is, long-term hospitalization and long-term psychotherapy (Stone 1998).

Adverse Selection

Potential health insurance enrollees differ significantly in risk for illness expense. Since the managed care marketplace rewards those health plans with the lowest treatment costs, all for-profit insurers try to avoid accepting responsibility for high-risk, expensive patients. They compete to attract primarily low-risk consumers by means of selective marketing and insuring (**risk selection**) (Herzlinger 1997; Kuttner 1998a; 1998b), shifting the costs of caring for the most ill and expensive patients to other plans (Kuttner 1998a). **Risk adjustment,** paying appropriately more for the treatment of severely ill patients, if it existed, would compensate for **adverse selection.** The absence of adequate risk adjustment creates serious financial risk for those providers caught with significant adverse selection (Newhouse 1994; Hacker 1997b; Chang et al. 1998).

Accurate determination of expected costs (financial risks) of particular populations of patients, the basis for risk adjustments of capitation payments, is not possible at present. Available risk adjustment models underpredict expenditures for patients with moderate and severe mental illness (Ettner and Notman 1997). Accurate mechanisms for mitigation of the consequences of adverse selection must be developed with appropriate adjustment of capitation or other reimbursement rates in order to protect the viability of providers who treat severely ill patients.

At present, the best solution for risk adjustment for expensive patients is the proposal of Newhouse (1993) and Ettner and Notman (1997:356) that payments "should not be fully capitated, but should involve some amount of risk-sharing on the part of the payer." **Partial-risk capitation** reduces risk of unexpected losses. It also "reduces the potential for a vendor to earn windfall profits" (Busch 1997:315). States and other payers have the power to dictate in partial-risk capitation contracts how much profit-taking is permissible. They also can require provision of a minimum number of services for certain diagnoses and/or levels of impairment (Busch 1997). **Full-risk capitation** exposes contractors to higher risks of financial loss but also to opportunity for higher profits. It maximizes their incentive to minimize resource expenditures. It encourages denying even appropriate and necessary care, which can easily be done because most payers mandate provision of benefit-package services only when medically necessary (Busch 1997). Mandated services must be available, but access to these services can be arbitrarily restricted. Full capitation is attractive to payers because it allows very accurate budgeting for health care costs (e.g., state Medicaid mental health costs). Regardless of the nature of contracts, however, private-sector contractees can be expected to shift costs wherever possible back to the public sector (Busch 1997).

The problem of adverse selection is especially relevant for public mental health providers. States tend to significantly underfund Medicaid managed behavioral health care programs, underestimating the cost of treating chronically and seriously mentally ill individuals, especially when access is made easier (Chang et al. 1998; Washington State 1998). The managed behavioral health care providers, having accepted underfunded, at-risk contracts (following a competitive bidding process), pay themselves for expensive administrative costs and allowed profits and then minimize their own risk exposure by subcontracting the care of moderately and severely ill patients to public mental health centers with inappropriately low, non-risk-adjusted, at-risk capitation rates (Chang et al. 1998). Moreover, responsibility for the care of the less severely ill Medicaid patients is retained by private providers, leaving the safety net public providers with higher proportions of expensive and uninsured patients. This adverse selection and absence of adequate risk adjustment leaves community-based mental health centers significantly under-reimbursed and at risk of bankruptcy. This severely disrupts the traditional, public safety net for persons with chronic mental illness (Busch 1997; Chang et al. 1998). The treatment needs of chronically mentally ill individuals, children and adults, must be protected by governmental funding that is adequate in amount and kept separate from funding for general medical care and the treatment of less severe psychiatric illness (Chang et al. 1998). **Psychiatric administrators must advocate strongly for the integrity of this funding.**

Principle 5: Physician and nonphysician practitioners constantly operate in a stressful environment of conflict of interest.

In the current managed care environment physicians are placed at significantly increased financial and legal risk for their treatment decisions. The financial incentive to minimize resource expenditure is pervasive (Hacker 1997b; Kuttner 1998a; 1998b). Physicians increasingly are paid on the basis of capitation, which encourages withholding treatment to increase organization profit and personal income (Kuttner 1998a; Stone 1998). A variety of other mechanisms are utilized to insure that physician income is substantially dependent upon withholding resource expenditure (Kuttner 1998a). To what extent are physicians able to work primarily on behalf of patient well-being, versus working in their personal financial self-interest, or versus working primarily in the interest of the fiscal security of their employers (Kassirer 1998; Stone 1998)? **There should be no financial incentives for physicians to deny appropriate and necessary care.**

Managed care insurers uniformly attempt to place the full burden of legal risk on their providers (Kuttner 1998b). Although consumer protection laws have been passed by many state legislatures during this decade permitting litigation against managed care plans over malpractice consequences of their clinical decisions (Kuttner 1998b; Sacks 1998), litigation is permissible only against plans lacking federal Employee Retirement Income Security Act (ERISA 1974) protection (Mariner 1996; Stone 1998). ERISA prohibits states from regulating the self-insured health plans of large employers and prevents patients from suing these managed care plans and corporations under state malpractice laws (Mariner 1996). Until Congress amends ERISA to permit states to regulate all managed care plans, most employer-funded, managed care insurers are free from liability (Stone 1998). What are the legal implications of denying reimbursement for health care? Every physician and hospital can be sued for malpractice. Should all involved decision-makers be legally responsible for malpractice consequences of denials of reimbursement? If not, ERISA, by removing risk of lawsuits on behalf of 120 million ERISA-covered individuals, will continue to lower the cost of malpractice to managed care insurers and markedly reduce the incentive to value patient well-being and physician professional integrity that arises from fear of malpractice litigation.

Physicians allocate a preponderance of health care resources. The cornerstone of managed care functioning is **control of medical decision making** such that the exercise of professional judgment is strongly constrained (Stone 1998). By inducing or forcing physicians to deny care they believe to be necessary, however, managed care insurers are attempting to redefine what constitutes medical necessity and acceptable standards of care. Physicians should always have autonomy to provide (at least minimally) necessary care for their ill patients, constrained where necessary by rationing imposed by society at large (**medical rationing is a societal moral dilemma, not a business profit or loss issue**). Otherwise, physicians become economic agents—employees of commercial enterprises operating for their own and for stockholder profit—no longer functioning primarily as members of a (once?) honored profession (Kassirer 1998; Stone 1998). The practice of medicine should not become "just another business" (Schroeder 1996). **Psychiatric administrators must advocate strongly for the integrity of appropriate professional autonomy.** They must work to optimize clinician authority and freedom to deal flexibly and creatively with patient problems.

Marmor identifies "loss of professional morale and patient trust" as dangers of managed care medicine's "bureaucratic and financial constraints on patient choice and physician judgment" (1998:563). Horton describes the "undermining of professional commitment" and the introduction of "the ethos . . . [and] values . . . of a business, not a service" as particularly destructive aspects of the Thatcher-era managed care–like administration of England's National Health Service (NHS): "doctors and nurses know that the changes in NHS culture have destroyed morale . . . (and led to) a fatal loss of goodwill . . . It is hard to forgive Thatcher for this" (Horton 1998:22). The profit-driven business ethos of American managed care that Sharfstein identifies as "corrupt at its core" must not be allowed to destroy the professional integrity and morale of medical and psychiatric practice (1998:21). **A primary goal of psychiatric administrators must be to effect change that improves clinician autonomy, professional identity and integrity, and morale.**

ACKNOWLEDGMENTS

Grateful acknowledgment is made to Robert F. Simpson, Bill J. Duke, Ph.D., Susan Schroeder, John Jamieson, M.D., and Sharon Ann Staton for valuable editorial suggestions and technical assistance.

GLOSSARY

Adverse selection The enrollment of a disproportionate number of high risk, expensive patients in a health insurance plan

Capitation payment A prospectively determined payment for all medically necessary covered health care services to be provided for one year for one health insurance plan enrollee

Cost shifting The process of shifting responsibility for payment of health care costs to another party

Discounted payments Reduced payment levels demanded by managed care insurer organizations

Discretionary costs Relatively unnecessary costs (for heath care) that can be incurred at will

Elastic demand Demand (for a health care product or service) that changes in magnitude in direct response to the personal cost of that product or service to the consumer

Fiduciary responsibility The obligation to provide expected benefits to investors or owners (of a health care business)

Fill-risk capitation Capitation payment (for health care services) that is contracted to be payment in full, regardless of expenses incurred (to provide these services)

Idemnity insurance Insurance that involves retrospective compensation for (health care) costs incurred

Medical-loss ratio The percentage of each health care premium dollar expended to provide patient care

Oligopolistic management Management or control of a market by only a few sellers

Partial-risk capitation A contract for health care service delivery that does not involve prospective payment in full but that includes some degree of ongoing responsibility for cost expenditures on the part of the payer

Price sensitive Higher out-of-pocket cost reduces overall consumer demand and payer expenditure

Privatization The process of contracting with private sector providers for services previously supplied by the public sector

Prospective payment A payment amount for health care service that is determined prospectively, before the service is delivered

Provider-sponsored organizations Networks of physician groups and hospitals that have developed the management capacity to contract directly with payer coalitions

Retrospective cost-based reimbursement The process of retrospectively paying charges for health care that are based upon the costs of the services delivered

Risk adjustment The process of paying providers appropriately more for the treatment of severely ill health plan enrollees

Risk selection The process of attracting low risk (low treatment cost) enrollees by selective marketing and insuring

Risk shifting The process of shifting the risk of health care financial losses to another party

Shadow buying The process whereby large managed care insurers cooperate to favorably price (for their own profit margins) their premium rates to employers

Vertical integration Ownership of multiple vertical business components, e.g., hospitals, physician groups, intermediate care facilities, etc.

Withholds Reimbursements for health care services that are withheld by health insurance plans and paid only if the providers meet specified performance expectations

REFERENCES

AFL-CIO. 1998. *Paying More and Losing Ground: How Employer Cost Shifting Is Eroding Health Coverage of Working Families.* Washington, DC: AFL-CIO.

AHA 1997. Section for Psychiatric and Substance Abuse Services. *Issues in Mental Health Coverage.* Chicago: American Hospital Association (AHA).

Analytical Perspectives. 1998. *Budget of the United States Government, Fiscal Year 1998.* Washington, DC: Office of Management and Budget.

Angell, M. 1997. Editorial: Fixing Medicare. *New England Journal of Medicine* 337:192–95.

Beinecke, K. H., and A. Lockhart. 1998. A provider assessment of the Massachusetts Medicaid managed behavioral health program: Year four. *Administration and Policy in Mental Health* 25:411–26.

Bodenheimer, T., and K. Sullivan. 1998a. How large employers are shaping the health care marketplace. First of two parts. *New England Journal of Medicine* 338:1003–7.

Bodenheimer, T., and K. Sullivan. 1998b. How large employers are shaping the health care marketplace. Second of two parts. *New England Journal of Medicine* 338:1084–87.

Busch, S. 1997. Carving-out mental health benefits to Medicaid beneficiaries: A shift toward managed care. *Administration and Policy in Mental Health* 24:301–21.

Chang, C. F., L. J. Kiser, J. E. Bailey, and M. Martins, et al. 1998. Tennessee's failed managed care program for mental health and substance abuse services. *Journal of the American Medical Association* 279:864–69.

Ellwood, P., Jr. 1997. An interview with Paul Ellwood, Jr., M.D. *Managed Care* 6 (11): 53–68.

Emery, B. D., R. W. Glover, and N. A. Mazade. 1998. The environmental trends facing state mental health agencies. *Administration and Policy in Mental Health* 25:337–47.

Employee Retirement Income Security Act of 1974. 1974. As amended, 29 U.S.C.: 1001–461.

Ettner, S. L., and E. H. Notman. 1997. How well do ambulatory care groups predict expenditures on mental health and substance abuse patients? *Administration and Policy in Mental Health* 24:339–57.

Foster Higgins. 1997. *National Survey of Employer-Sponsored Health Plans 1996.* New York: William Mercer.

Foster Higgins. 1998. *National Survey of Employer-Sponsored Health Plans 1997.* New York, NY: William Mercer.

Gabel, J. 1997. Ten ways HMOs have changed during the 1990s. *Health Affairs* 16 (3): 134–45.

Ginsberg, P. B., and J. D. Pickreign. 1996. Tracking health care costs. *Health Affairs* 15 (5): 140–49.

Ginzberg, E., and M. Ostow. 1997. Managed care—A look back and a look ahead. *New England Journal of Medicine* 336:1018–20.

Goldman, W., J. McCulloch, and R. Sturm. 1998. Costs and use of mental health services before and after managed care. *Health Affairs* 17 (2): 40–52.

Gramm, P., A. J. Rettenmaier, and T. R. Saving. 1998a. Medicare policy for future generations—A search for a permanent solution. *New England Journal of Medicine* 338:1307–10.

Gramm, P., A. J. Rettenmaier, and T. R. Saving. 1998b. Letter to the editor. Reforming Medicare: The Gramm plan. *New England Journal of Medicine* 339:778.

Hacker, J. S. 1997a. *The Road to Nowhere: The Genesis of President Clinton's Plan for Health Security.* Princeton, NJ: Princeton University Press.

Hacker, J. S. 1997b. Book review: Market-driven health care. *Journal of Health Politics, Policy and Law* 22:1443–48.

Hay Group. 1998. *Health Care Plan Design and Cost Trends—1988 through 1997.* Washington, DC: National Association of Psychiatric Health Systems.

Herzlinger, R. E. 1997. *Market-Driven Health Care: Who Wins, Who Loses in the Transformation of America's Largest Service Industry.* Reading, MA: Addison-Wesley.

Hilzenrath, D. S. 1997. Finding something left to squeeze: Managed-care firms discover costs are rising and cuts are getting harder to come by. *Washington Post National Weekly Edition,* 14 July, 20–21.

Hodgkin, D., C. M. Horgan, and D. W. Garnick. 1997. Make or buy: HMOs' contracting arrangements for mental health care. *Administration and Policy in Mental Health* 24:359–76.

Horton, R. 1998. A revision of expectations. *London Review of Books,* 20 (13): 20–22.

Iglehart, J. K. 1997. Listening in on the Duke University Private Sector Conference. *New England Journal of Medicine* 336:1827–31.

Iglehart, J. K. 1998. Medicare and graduate medical education. *New England Journal of Medicine* 338:402–7.

Kassirer, J. P. 1995. Editorial: Managed care and the morality of the marketplace. *New England Journal of Medicine* 333:50–52.

Kassirer, J. P. 1997. Editorial: Is managed care here to stay? *New England Journal of Medicine* 336:1013–14.

Kassirer, J. P. 1998. Editorial: Managing care—Should we adopt a new ethic? *New England Journal of Medicine* 339:397–98.

Kuttner, R. 1998a. Must good HMOs go bad? The commercialization of prepaid group health care. *New England Journal of Medicine* 338:1558–63.

Kuttner, R. 1998b. Must good HMOs go bad? The search for checks and balances. *New England Journal of Medicine* 338:1635–39.

Larkin, H. 1996. Employed but uninsured: Why business is cutting back on health insurance. *Robert Wood Johnson Foundation Advances* 1:1–5.

Latham, S. R. 1996. Regulation of managed care incentive payments to physicians. *American Journal of Law and Medicine* 4:399–432.

Levit, K. R., H. C. Lazenby, C. A. Cowan, and D. K. Won. 1995. State health expenditure accounts: Building blocks for state health spending analysis. *Health Care Financing Review* 17:201–54.

Libby, A. M. 1997. Contracting between public and private providers: A survey of mental health services in California. *Administration and Policy in Mental Health* 24:323–38.

Lynch, F. L. 1997. The effects of state intergovernmental transfers on local public mental health services. *Administration and Policy in Mental Health* 24:279–99.

Managed care now "firmly in control" but its final shape remains in question. 1998. *Psychiatric News* 33 (5): 1, 30.

Mariner, W. K. 1996. State regulation of managed care and the Employee Retirement Income Security Act. *New England Journal of Medicine* 335:1986–90.

Marmor, T. R. 1998. Forecasting American health care: How we got here and where we might be going. *Journal of Health Politics, Policy and Law* 23:551–71.

McKusick, D., T. L. Mark, E. King, R. Harwood, J. A. Buck, J. Dilonardo, and J. S. Genuardi. 1998. Spending for mental health and substance abuse treatment, 1996. *Health Affairs* 17 (4): 9–21.

Moran, G. F. 1998. The economics of care. *Minnesota Physician* 11 (1): 1, 10–11, 37.

Morgan, R. O., B. A. Virnig, C. A. DeVito, and N. A. Persily. 1997. The Medicare-HMO revolving door—The healthy go in and the sick go out. *New England Journal of Medicine* 337:169–75.

National Association of Psychiatric Health Systems (NAPHS). 1997. *1997 Annual Survey Report.* Washington, DC: NAPHS.

NAPHS 1997 annual survey reports trends. 1997. *Business Wire,* 8 September, 1–2.

Naylor, C. D. 1995. Grey zones of clinical practice: Some limits to evidence-based medicine. *Lancet* 345:840–42.

Naylor, C. D. 1998. Editorial: What is appropriate care? *New England Journal of Medicine* 338:1918–20.

Newhouse, J. P. 1993. *Free for All.* Cambridge, MA: Harvard University Press.

Office of the Chief Economist. 1996. *A Look at Employers' Costs of Providing Health Benefits.* Washington, DC: U.S. Department of Labor, 31 July 1996.

Patterson, D. Y. 1993. What percentage of premium should HMOs allocate for behavioral healthcare? *Behavioral Healthcare Tomorrow* 2 (5): 27–28.

Pearson, S. D., J. E. Sabin, and E. J. Emanuel. 1998. Ethical guidelines for physician compensation based on capitation. *New England Journal of Medicine* 339:689–93.

Physician Payment Review Commission. 1996a. *Arrangements between Managed Care Plans and Physicians. II. A Follow-up on the Analysis of 1994 Survey Data and Site Visit Information.* Washington, DC: Physician Payment Review Commission, June.

Physician Payment Review Commission. 1996b. *How Do Plans Pay Network Physicians?* Washington, DC: Physician Payment Review Commission, November.

Relman, A. S. 1998. Book review: The economic future of health care. *New England Journal of Medicine* 338:1855–56.

Rettig, R. A. 1994. Medical innovation duels cost containment. *Health Affairs* 13 (3): 7–27.
Rettig, R. A. 1997. *Health Care in Transition: Technology Assessment in the Private Sector.* Santa Monica, CA: Rand.
Robinson, J. C. 1994. The changing boundaries of the American hospital. *Milbank Quarterly* 72:259–75.
Sacks, H. S. 1998. Managed care is feeling sick. *Psychiatric News,* 6 March, 3, 32.
Samuelson, R. J. 1996. The Medicaid morass. *Washington Post National Weekly Edition,* 19 February, 5.
Schroeder, S. A. 1996. The triumph of the market: What does it bode for health and health care? *Robert Wood Johnson Foundation Annual Report,* 7–20. Princeton, NJ.
Schroeder, S. A. 1997. Informing debate: A private role in public issues. *Robert Wood Johnson Foundation Annual Report,* 6–17. Princeton, NJ.
Sharfstein, S. S. 1998. A radical solution to managed care woes. *Psychiatric News* 33:17, 21.
Shortell, S. M., R. R. Gillies, and K. J. Devers. 1995. Reinventing the American hospital. *Milbank Quarterly* 73:131–60.
Smith, B. M. 1997. Trends in health care coverage and financing and their implications for policy. *New England Journal of Medicine* 337:1000–1003.
Staton, D. 1989. Mental health care economics and the future of psychiatric practice. *Psychiatric Annals* 19:421–27.
Stoeckle, J. D. 1995. The citadel cannot hold: Technologies go outside the hospital, patients and doctors too. *Milbank Quarterly* 73:3–17.
Stone, A. A. 1998. Market forces: The iceberg to medicine's Titanic. *Psychiatric Times* 15 (10): 23–29.
Struss, V., and K. J. Halleland. 1998. A new opportunity: Provider sponsored organizations come to Minnesota. *Minnesota Physician* 11 (10): 12–13, 28.
Sturm, R. 1997. How expensive is unlimited mental health care coverage under managed care? *Journal of the American Medical Association* 278:1533–37.
Sturm, R., and J. McCulloch. 1998. Mental health and substance abuse benefits in carve-out plans and the Mental Health Parity Act of 1996. *Journal of Health Care Finance* 24 (3): 82–92.
Thorpe, K. E. 1997. The health system in transition: Care, cost, and coverage. *Journal of Health Politics, Policy and Law* 22:339–61.
Ware, J. E., Jr., M. S. Bayliss, W. H. Rogers, M. Kosinski, and A. R. Tarlov. 1996. Differences in 4-year health outcomes for elderly and poor, chronically ill patients treated in HMO and fee-for-service systems: Results from the Medical Outcomes Study. *Journal of the American Medical Association* 276:1039–47.
Washington Business Group on Health (WBGH). 1996. *Recent Trends in Private Sector Mental Health Strategies.* Washington, DC: WBGH.
Washington State terminates Medicaid managed care. 1998. *Psychiatric News* 33 (2): 1, 32.

CHAPTER 2

Mental Health Care Delivery Systems

Kenneth Gaver, M.D.

Mental health care delivery systems are constantly evolving and changing in response to a variety of forces, many of which are succinctly described in chapter 1 of this book. **Systems in existence today may vary greatly in the coming years as economic and societal forces and advancing technologies render the present forms obsolete.**

This chapter describes the main mental health delivery systems currently operating. **These systems are often integral parts of or supported by other systems of social, economic, and supportive nature** that are too complex to describe in this chapter but of which mental health administrators should be cognizant.

Delivery systems also overlap one another. Public mental health systems may be based in local community, city, county, state, or federal agencies yet be directed by or financially dependent upon another level of authority. For example, county-based community mental health programs may be operated in accordance with state authority and funding. Private systems often contract with governmental agencies and vice versa. This renders the classification of systems difficult.

If one were describing only clinical systems, one might discuss them in traditional terms such as inpatient, partial hospitalization, day-care, outpatient, residential treatment, group homes, etc. But because the administrative settings in which such services are sited have significant requirements that vary greatly, it may be most convenient to describe mental health systems in terms of the administrative organization rather than clinical programs.

Overall Trends

The trends in delivery of mental health services are described in great detail (Redick et al. 1996). There has been a large decline in the numbers of hospitals, numbers of beds, admissions, and patient days in state mental hospitals. The number of admissions to psychiatric units of non-federal general hospitals and private psychiatric hospitals has markedly increased. Veterans hospitals' admissions have stayed fairly constant. Admissions to residential treatment centers have significantly increased. **Overall, the locus of patient care episodes has shifted from inpatient to outpatient.** In 1955, 77 percent were inpatient and 23 percent outpatient. By 1971 this had shifted to 42 percent and 55 percent, respectively, and by 1992 to 26 percent and 68 percent. The number of mental health organizations in the United States also increased from 3,005 in 1970 to 5,498 in 1992 (Redick et al. 1996).

Another major impact not readily reflected in the patient care episode statistics has been the enormous increase in managed care organizations affecting mental health care. These services typically aim to reduce patient days in hospital and emphasize ambulatory care. Currently, more than 120 million persons are now covered by private managed behavioral healthcare insurance plans (Manderscheid and Henderson 1996). As of 1996, "a total of twenty-two states had received federal waivers to implement managed behavioral health care programs" for Medicaid financed public mental health programs.

The private office practices of mental health practitioners are not reflected in the outpatient statistics, but do represent a portion of the managed care episodes and account for a high volume of admissions to non-federal general hospitals and private psychiatric hospitals.

Private Practice

Private office-based practice is probably the setting in which most mental health professionals practice. Such practices may be organized in many ways, the most frequent being solo practice, practice in small groups, or association with a psychiatrist, psychologist, social worker, or other professionals. Psychiatric practice in a multi-specialty medical group is another common format.

Most office-based practitioners also work in one or more settings besides the office. This may include inpatient or partial hospitalization services in an acute care or psychiatric hospital, a residential treatment center, or a clinic. Many practitioners also have contractual or part-time appointments in community mental health programs, court or jail services, schools, teaching institutions, nursing homes, or other sites. Each of these sites may have its own unique expectations for clinical practice and administrative procedures.

Outpatient private practice today is driven by the requirements of the payer as well as the clinical needs of the patient. Most practitioners, in order

to survive, must be a member of panels of providers controlled by the payer, whether it be an indemnity insurance company, a Health Maintenance Organization (HMO), a Behavioral Healthcare Organization (BHO), a Preferred Provider Organization (PPO), or an Independent Practice Association (IPA). Medicare and Medicaid also have clinical and administrative requirements. Just filing of claims for payment represents a major administrative task. Many organizations also require that a treatment plan be developed, approved, and periodically reviewed and revised. Many managed care organizations also have treatment protocols or guidelines that must be adhered to. Furthermore, managed care organizations may require site visits of the office to review records and practices.

Administration of an office-based or group practice thus becomes much more complicated. The usual tasks of acquiring, furnishing, supplying and staffing an office, scheduling patients, recording billing and collecting charges, maintaining insurance, marketing, keeping and recording medical records, etc., are the minimum. A group practice may have contracts with payers or membership on multiple, perhaps dozens or hundreds, of insurance panels. Each contract must be monitored for special requirements, payment rates, and schedules and must be continuously reviewed to ensure the validity and renewability of the contract. Multiple billing procedures are required and collection and aging of accounts is necessary.

One of the great pitfalls of membership on provider panels is the possibility of removal from the panel. Payers may remove providers for many reasons, such as too many panelists, arbitrary limits on number of visits, failure to follow protocols, etc. Survivability as a practitioner then demands that all contracts be systematically monitored.

Large multiple specialty groups may have unique problems. There may be competition for space and staff, problems in coordinating care among the many specialists, etc. It is not unusual for friction to exist among thc various specialties regarding income differences (e.g., revenue per provider). Unfortunately, mental health services score low in this category compared to surgeons, radiologists, or anaesthesiologists.

From this, **it is clear that office-based private practice has its own unique set of administrative challenges.**

Acute Care (General) Hospitals

The most important mental health components of acute care hospitals are emergency rooms, scatter beds, and psychiatric units. To a lesser extent, acute care hospitals may provide partial hospitalization and outpatient services.

The importance of the emergency room in providing emergency psychiatric evaluations cannot be underestimated. While there are no hard figures available, **the emergency rooms of acute care hospitals provide a vast amount of emergency and triage services in mental health.** In many communities this may be the primary locus of emergency and triage mental health services.

Since most emergency rooms are staffed by physicians and nurses specializing in emergency medicine, the evaluation and disposition of mental health patients is often provided by contractual arrangements with mental health organizations or practitioners in the community. If an organized community mental health program exists, it is common practice to contract with that program for provision of mental health services in the emergency room on an on-call basis with staff specifically trained and available for such purposes. Most often, these are clinicians from psychology, social work, or counseling backgrounds. A psychiatrist is usually available for backup. If the acute care hospital operates a special psychiatric unit, then staff from the unit will often provide the service in the emergency room. Again, an on-call psychiatrist should be available for consultation and to arrange for hospital admission.

The emergency room staff and the mental health clinicians must be provided with guidelines for the prioritization of patient services and diagnostic, decision, and referral guidelines. They must also have knowledge of extensive resources in the community ranging from inpatient to outpatient and social support agencies and self-help groups. Administrative and clinical guidance must be provided. It may be wise also for an experienced clinician to occasionally audit services to ensure the reliability of diagnoses, decisions, and referrals.

Scatter beds are those general medical-surgical beds that may be available for a mental health patient. Most often, such patients are cared for by the attending physician. Again, there is a high volume of such patients in acute care hospitals, as many as 500,000 admissions per year (Redick et al. 1996). These tend most often to be patients not overtly dangerous to themselves or others and not in severe acute psychiatric crisis. There may be a high degree of comorbidity with medical/surgical conditions. There is no reliable estimate of the number of scatter beds since these are not dedicated mental health beds. **Probably the most important clinical/administrative issue is the provision of an adequate system of consultation-liaison services to support the attending physician and to ensure appropriate referral when indicated.**

Organized psychiatric units are frequent components of acute care hospitals. As of 1992, there were 1,616 non-federal acute care hospitals with separate psychiatric services of which 1,517 provided inpatient services (Redick et al. 1996). These services provided 52,049 psychiatric beds and accounted for 46 percent of all inpatient admissions in the United States. Two hundred eighteen units also provided outpatient care providing 14.9 percent of outpatient admissions while 423 provided partial care with 17.9 percent of admissions (Redick et al. 1996).

Such units may range in size from just a few beds with medical and nursing care and few ancillary services to large, well-organized services with a full range of ancillary services. Most commonly, they will have primary medical and nursing care and at least some ancillary services. They may also provide day treatment and outpatient care. Most admissions are of short duration, e.g., six to ten days, and the most common aftercare resource is the attending physician. Some allow admissions by non-physician clinicians with co-physician care. Most require admitting privileges reserved to psychiatrists or other mental health clinicians. A few allow admission by any attending physician. Acute care hospitals may also offer specialty psychiatric services to children, adolescents, the geriatric patient, or to patients with medical and psychiatric comorbidity (medical-psychiatric units). They may also offer alcohol or substance abuse services.

The larger, well-organized psychiatric units present administrative issues similar to those discussed later under private psychiatric hospitals. The less intensive units usually will have a part-time, contracted psychiatrist as a medical director. **The administrative issues often revolve around the financial viability of the unit.** The average daily occupancy for units under twelve beds may not be economically feasible, given staffing requirements and reimbursement.

Large psychiatric units of acute care hospitals generally require an executive officer who is an intimate member of the overall hospital executive team. Most will require a part-time to half-time medical director and many will require a director of psychiatric nursing. Program or clinical directors for special units may also be needed. Familiarity with the Special Conditions for Psychiatric Hospitals in the Medicare Conditions of Participation and special issues for psychiatric services in the contemporary Joint Commission on Accreditation of Healthcare Organization's (JCAHO) *Comprehensive Accreditation Manual for Hospitals* (JCAHO 1998) **are essential for the proper management of the unit.** Some state hospital licensing regulations may also have specific requirements for such units. **Other administrative issues will reflect medical staff organization, quality assurance, utilization review, the quality of medical records, and patient safety.**

Private Psychiatric Hospitals

Private psychiatric hospitals were a growth industry in the last two decades. There were 184 private psychiatric hospitals in 1980, increasing to 475 by 1992. The number of inpatient beds rose from 17,157 to 43,684 during that same period. Admissions rose from 140,381 in 1979 to 467,827 in 1992 and represented 24 percent of inpatient and residential care episodes nationally (Redick et al. 1997).

Private psychiatric hospitals have been in existence in the United States since the latter part of the eighteenth century. The great growth in the last few decades came with increased fee-for-service reimbursement. Many corporations emerged as for-profit operators of multi-hospital chains. Enormous growth occurred in the care of children and adolescents with specialty programs dedicated to these and other groups.

The number, size, and length of stay of patients have been greatly attenuated by the advent of managed care. As a result, the private psychiatric hospitals have been reducing their numbers, size, and length of stay. Increasingly, they have diversified their services to provide partial hospitalization, residential, and outpatient care and have contracted to become affiliated with HMOs and PPOs.

In 1933 the National Association of Private Psychiatric Hospitals (NAPPH) was formed to represent these organizations. That organization is now named the National Association of Psychiatric Health Systems (NAPHS) and now offers membership to organizations other than private psychiatric hospitals. The NAPHS Annual Survey Report 1997 (NAPHS 1997) indicates that 90 percent of its 316 members were private psychiatric hospitals, 5 percent general hospital psychiatric units, and 4 percent residential treatment centers. In 1996, 17.6 percent of its members were not-for-profit organizations, 4.7 percent independent (for-profit), and 77.9 percent were multi-facility for-profit facilities.

For-profit hospitals typically are organized, like acute care hospitals, with an independent medical and professional staff whose income is derived from patient-care billings rather than the hospital itself. It is more common for not-for-profit hospitals to have a professional staff that derives a portion, if not most, of its income from the hospital and the rest from patient care billings. **Both types will generally have both full-time administrative executives and a medical director, occasionally full-time but more often part-time, compensated from the hospital by salary or contract. Most will also have part-time clinical or program directors from medical or other disciplines to be responsible for the clinical care in specialty programs.**

Special programs vary widely according to interests of the staff and the needs of the community. In addition to adult inpatient services and children's and/or adolescents' services, they may also include specialty programs such as addiction disorders, sexual dysfunction disorders, geriatric programs, etc. Increasingly, most hospitals have partial hospitalization programs, outpatient services, and residential treatment.

The volume of private psychiatric hospital care is illustrated by the following figures for 1992 (Redick et al. 1996).

	Number	*Percentage of All U.S.*
Inpatient additions	469,827	22.5
Outpatient additions	140,824	4.9
Partial care additions	65,354	23.1

NAPHS, with 239 of its 316 member facilities reporting, estimated 476,844 inpatient admissions in its 295 hospitals with 24,780 set up and staffed beds. The number of days of care is progressively declining for each episode of care as illustrated by the following (NAPHS 1997):

	1993	*1994*	*1995*	*1996*
Inpatient length of stay (days)	16.2	16.4	11.7	11.5
Average number partial hospitalization visits			17	13
Average number outpatient visits		22.5	15.4	8.7

Private hospitals in 1996 derived 46.3 percent of their revenues from Medicare, Medicaid and the Civilian Health and Medical Program for the Uniformed Services (CHAMPUS), 24.7 percent from HMOs and PPOs, and 17.5 percent from commercial insurance, the remainder being from a variety of other sources.

Many of the administrative issues in private psychiatric hospitals parallel those in acute care hospital psychiatric units including issues relating to state licensing, Medicare certification, JCAHO accreditation, utilization review, and quality assurance and improvement. The administrator and medical director personnel, however, have special duties relating to governance, medical staff bylaws and rules and regulations, defining clinical privileges and granting and updating practitioner competence for clinical privileges, hospital administrative and clinical policies and procedures, the oversight of an often elaborate range of ancillary services, etc. Furthermore, the medical director often must exercise considerable diplomacy in managing the intrastaff tensions and conflicts and the relationship between an independent medical staff and the hospital administration.

Finally, as managed care delivery organizations continue to expand, private hospitals are increasingly contracting with such organizations to deliver services. Sixty-six percent of the 1997 survey respondents were part of one or more managed care networks (NAPHS 1977). Additional contracts involved employers, community programs, and contracts with state mental health authorities. **The need for contract monitoring and management is growing and can be expected to continue growth.**

State Mental Health Authorities

State Mental Health Authorities (SMHAs) are those components of state government that have the legal responsibility to operate or fund mental health services with state revenues within each state. Traditionally, such services have included state mental hospitals and state-sponsored community mental health programs. They may be free-standing departments of state government or components of other state human resource agencies. They may administer federally funded programs and must work collaboratively with other state agencies, particularly the agencies that administer Medicaid funds, health agencies, and social services. **The range of administrative responsibilities may be very broad and complex.**

State Mental Health Authorities may also operate, fund, or oversee numerous other programs as illustrated by the *FY96 SMHA Profiling System, Narrative Highlights* published by the National Association of State Mental Health Program Directors Research Institute, Inc. (NASMHPD 3). That publication describes the major programs of the District of Columbia and forty-eight of the fifty states, Mississippi and South Dakota being excepted. Of the forty-nine jurisdictions covered, all are the SMHAs. They also have the responsibility for alcoholism and drug dependency in twenty states, mental retardation in eighteen states, and developmental disabilities other than mental retardation in twelve states. Twenty-four of the SMHAs have the responsibility for forensic mental health services while thirteen share that responsibility for other agencies. Mental health services in state correctional facilities are usually the responsibility of the corrections agencies often with SMHA collaboration except that in at least five states, the SMHA has the responsibility. Some SMHAs also have the responsibility for the licensing of private psychiatric hospitals.

State Mental Hospitals

State mental hospitals have been a traditional responsibility of SMHAs, but it should be noted that a few counties have the equivalent of state mental hospitals. With deinstitutionalization and decentralization of services, the role of state mental hospitals is declining. In 1970 there were 310 such hospitals with 369,969 resident patients. By 1992 the number had declined to 273 with 83,180 patients. During that same period the number of additions had declined from 486,661 to 275,382 or a drop from 37.9 percent to

13.2 percent of all national additions (Redick et al. 1996). Since 1992 the SMHAs have continued to close or to decrease the size of state mental hospitals. There are many fewer today and even more will be closed in the future (NASMHPD 1996).

State mental hospitals continue to play a role in the care of those patients who are so chronically and severely ill as to constitute a danger to themselves or others and for those patients identified as forensic (i.e., not guilty by reason of insanity or not competent to stand trial). Many state hospitals also serve special populations such as sex offenders. They may also operate programs that may not be feasibly operated by community mental health agencies including, for example, services for mentally disordered juvenile offenders. Some state hospitals operate partial hospital and outpatient programs.

In past years the chief executive officer was usually a physician. That practice has largely been replaced with a professional administrator and a medical director. Program or clinical directors may supervise units or programs. Most hospitals are Medicare certified and JCAHO accredited although outmoded physical plants may negate both possibilities.

Community Mental Health Programs

The number and variety of community mental health programs is staggering. Many such programs were initiated by state governments prior to the passage of the Community Mental Health Centers Act of 1963 (CMHC 1963). Thus, while influenced by the federal act, they have evolved in those directions necessary to meet the priorities of the SMHAs and the needs of the communities.

The number of additions to community mental health programs is probably the largest proportion of all additions to all services in the United States. They are included under the heading for all other organizations (Redick et al. 1996). That inclusive grouping represented 1,613 organizations in 1992, 520 of which had inpatient services, 1,309 had outpatient services, and 1,434 had partial care. They represented, however, 178,815 inpatient admissions, or 8.5 percent of the United States' total, but 1,544,776 outpatient additions, or 53.2 percent of the United States' total, far outweighing any other classification of organizations. They also represented 57.2 percent of partial care additions.

Most community mental health programs are operated or contracted by local governmental or quasi-governmental agencies. Services may be actually delivered by a variety of local governmental, quasi-governmental, not-for-profit or even for-profit agencies and through contracts with local hospitals and practitioners.

The majority provide a range of services including emergency psychiatric care, outpatient, inpatient, and day care along with case-finding and preventive and counseling services. They may include residential care and often a range of supportive service such as group homes, assisted living, dedicated housing, and housing assistance. Case management for the severely impaired is a fundamental service in many programs.

While community mental health programs often originated as outpatient services or mental health services for children, their focus has changed to provide services to the chronically and severely mentally ill including children, adolescents, and adults. The decline in state mental hospital populations and mandates from SMHAs to provide care for such persons have been major factors in this shift.

The sources of financial support for community mental health programs are numerous. Most state funding systems require some local match from local governmental resources. Medicaid reimbursement is a major factor. Some reimbursement is obtained from insurance sources and from managed care programs. But for most programs, SMHA funding is crucial. Of the forty-nine SMHAs (NASMHPD 1996), all of them reported a method of funding for local mental health programs using a variety of different methods based on the population served, the types of programs, and the priorities of the SMHAs. SMHAs often reported that the greatest percentage of funds controlled by SMHAs were for community mental health programs, for example, 83 percent in Alabama and Arizona, 73 percent in California, 43 percent in Alaska, ranging down to 25 percent in Montana and 22 percent in Nebraska (NASMHPD 1996).

Many SMHAs reported funding to a large number of local organizations including 126 in Illinois, 138 in New York, 175 in Ohio, all 57 counties in California, down to 13 in Idaho, and 3 in Nevada (NASMHPD 1996). The various community mental health programs being funded by SMHAs included at least 310 residential treatment centers for children and 219 acute care hospital psychiatric services. Community mental health programs are often funded by SMHAs to provide mental health services in local jails and correctional facilities.

In recent years SMHAs and their corresponding Medicaid agencies have undertaken to revamp their Medicaid programs to implement managed care by applying for 1915B or 1115 waivers. By 1995 at least forty states had received waivers (Stroup and Dowart 1997). These have included mainstreaming and carve-out programs. **Some states have contracted with a single managed care organization to manage the programs but most have utilized two or more organizations or even multiple organizations.**

Since a large proportion of traditional community mental health clien-

tele are eligible for services under Medicaid, the implication of Medicaid waivers for such programs is obvious. New organizational arrangements may be required, different services may be given priority and new organizations may be involved. Yet, since both the SMHAs and the community mental health programs share the responsibility for these clients, **it is clear that most of the services will be delivered by community mental health programs.**

Community programs also must meet the performance expectations of the SMHAs. They may also be expected to meet accreditation requirements relevant to community mental health programs that are available from the Joint Commission on Accreditation of Healthcare Organizations (JCAHO 1999), the Commission on Accreditation of Rehabilitation Facilities (CARF 1998), and the National Committee for Quality Assurance (NCQA 1997).

The variety of services offered, the multiple funding sources, the relationships with multiple levels of government, the organizational alternatives, and the characteristics of the clientele served make the administration of community programs challenging.

Department of Veterans Affairs

Potentially any veteran is eligible for mental health services from the many hospitals and clinics operated by the Department of Veterans Affairs. In practice most do not use the services since mental health care is available through other services and reimbursement mechanisms available to them. Furthermore, the department operates under a policy that those veterans who have a disability related to military service have priority access to care. Since the numbers of individuals engaged in military service fluctuates widely depending on military conflicts, the numbers of veterans with such service related disabilities also fluctuates. The residual number of veterans of the huge number of military personnel during World War II and now part of the geriatric population still generates a significant portion of veterans. This means that geriatric medical and mental health problems are significant in veterans facilities.

The number of Veterans Affairs Medical Centers that are mental health organizations has ranged from 115 in 1970 to 162 in 1992 (Redick et al. 1996). Those with inpatient mental health services have grown in that same period from 110 to 133, with outpatient services from 100 to 161, and with partial care services from 100 to 161. At the same time, the number of inpatient beds has declined from 50,688 in 1970 to 22,466 in 1992, the latter representing 8.5 percent of all U.S. beds. The total inpatient population has declined from 51,696 in 1970 to 18,531 in 1992 even as total additions increased from 135,216 to 180,529. **The main growth in mental health ser-**

vices to veterans has been in outpatient settings where additions increased from 16,790 in 1969 to 144,591 in 1992 with a similar increase in additions to partial care (Redick et al. 1996).

The Department of Veterans Affairs provides mental health services in its acute care hospitals and a few veterans psychiatric hospitals. It operates many outpatient clinics and partial care programs as well as alternative care services such as care in nursing homes.

For several decades, veterans medical centers have been built in conjunction with university medical schools and other training programs for allied health professionals. They are most closely allied with academic programs and serve an important function as teaching institutions. Medical center staff members thus have the opportunity to participate in teaching, research, and other academic pursuits as a result of this proximity. The medical centers conversely benefit from the advances in medical science and teaching thus so readily available.

The very nature of the population served by veterans facilities offers some unique clinical opportunities including geriatric problems, post-traumatic stress syndrome, mental health disorder with comorbidity with chronic illness and chronicity. Although still heavily weighted toward males, the increased number of females entering military service has created more opportunities for dealing with women than in previous years.

Since veterans programs' staff members are federal employees, they receive the benefits of such employment including health care, retirement, and other amenities. **On the other hand, administrative practices must be in conformance with those of a large bureaucracy.**

Department of Defense

The United States military forces provide medical care not only in the United States but in all countries where military troops are stationed. Mental health services are included in such services for active duty personnel, their dependents and, when practicable, for retired military personnel in the area.

Military acute care hospitals are available in many locations in the United States and abroad. Many acute care hospitals provide short-term mental health care in both scatter beds and in small inpatient units as well as outpatient units. Large military hospitals such as the National Naval Medical Center in Bethesda, MD, and the Walter Reed Army Medical Center have major psychiatric units as do other large military hospitals.

Smaller military bases do not generally have acute care hospitals but may have a dispensary with some short-stay acute care beds and outpatient services. Inpatient mental health services are not generally included but some ambulatory mental health services are provided. Major training bases usually have mental health services as essential to the screening and assessment of trainees as well as for ambulatory care. These will also be linked to acute care hospitals for more intensive evaluation and treatment.

During active military conflict mental health services are deployed as close to active combat as feasible to allow for triage, assessment, and short-term treatment of psychiatric casualties.

Since military facilities are linked by a worldwide transportation system, transfers from combat locations or from smaller military installations makes use of centralized mental health facilities much more feasible.

With the increased numbers of women in military service, the diversity of behavioral health programs has increased. In addition, military mental health services provide care to the spouses and the children of military personnel and to eligible military retirees who are in the area.

Long-term care of the mentally impaired retiree is provided by the Department of Veterans Affairs through its multitude of mental health resources. CHAMPUS provides care to many military retirees and their family members through contractual arrangements with civilian programs.

The statistical report, *Mental Health, United States, 1996* (Redick et al. 1996), does not include additions to inpatient, partial care, residential care, or outpatient care for the Department of Defense programs so that information is not included when statistical information is provided about other mental health organizations in this chapter.

Clinical issues in military mental health include the full range of clinical conditions except that the chronically and severely mentally impaired are less well represented. On the other hand, conditions related to long absences from home and family and the potential for post-traumatic stress syndrome may be more likely.

The administration of mental health services in military settings is modified by the expectations of military protocol and procedures. More exacting standards prevail in the screening and assessment of personnel than in most civilian settings. A career in the military forces usually ends at a period of time when a much longer professional life can be expected, thus requiring a change in circumstances and practice for mental health professionals who retire from military service.

Corrections Facilities

Corrections facilities include jails and prisons. The former are generally under local jurisdictions such as cities and counties, while prisons are operated by state departments of corrections and the Federal Bureau of Prisons. There are a few privately operated prisons. These facilities encounter many mentally ill persons and provide varied programs ranging from screening, identification, treatment, and diversion programs to outpatient, protected living, and inpatient care in prisons.

Correctional mental health is one of the most enigmatic but rapidly growing areas of mental health services. The reference material on the subject is sparse in professional mental health publications. Publications in the corrections literature and in government reports is a rich source of material. Resources, such as the National Institute of Corrections of the U.S. Department of Justice and the Center for Mental Health Services, Substance Abuse and Mental Health Services Administration, U.S. Department of Health and Human Services, are vital in obtaining information about mental health services in jails and prisons.

Most jails are small and lengths of stay in jail are a few days for most inmates. Screening, crisis intervention, and emergency care are the more frequently provided services. Many diversion programs exist specifically targeted toward persons who are arrested for misdemeanors or nonviolent crimes and who could benefit from local treatment services. **Such diversion programs are most frequently offered under contracts or agreements with local community mental health programs.** There is also a group of prisoners admitted under felony charges who may have chronic and severe mental illness often with comorbid substance abuse and a history of non-compliance with mental health treatment. **Some larger jails offer special units to care for these persons since they are generally not candidates for diversion programs.** Suicide is a prominent risk in both jails and prisons and may rank as the number one cause of death in corrections facilities. Over half of suicides in jails occur within the first day of admission and over one-fourth of them within the first three hours (Rowen and Hayes 1995). They are most frequent among mentally ill persons, many of whom communicate their intent and may have made previous attempts (DuRand et al. 1995).

The magnitude of the problem of the mentally ill in jails is illustrated in a review of the literature since 1970 (Lamb and Weinberger 1998). **The authors summarize findings that by 1995 there were more than 483,000 persons in jails and that between 6 and 15 percent suffered serious mental disorders.**

Prisons, in contrast to jails, tend to be large facilities whose inmates remain for protracted periods. **In 1995 there were more than 1,587,000 inmates of state and federal prisons of whom an estimated 10 to 15 percent suffered severe mental illness** (Lamb and Weinberger 1998). The mentally ill populations of prisons thus exceeds that of state mental hospitals. These estimates do not include the thousands of forensic patients mostly cared for by SMHAs.

Persons in prisons are often identified as having suffered mental illness prior to incarceration. There is a significant comorbidity with substance abuse. Many have been resistant to prior treatment. The majority of prisons offer some mental health treatment including individual therapy, group therapy, psychoactive medication, and a variety of supportive programs, particularly those targeted to chemical dependence. Psychologists, social workers, and non-professionally trained mental health workers constitute the majority of staff with psychiatrists generally being in short supply. Many prisoners are housed within the general prison populations, but some prisons offer mental health programs that include residential living and even acute hospital care. Relationships among corrections agencies and SMHAs are variable. In a few states SMHAs assume responsibility for the mental health programs but in the majority of states, services, except perhaps for hospital care, are provided through employees or contract staff in the correctional agencies. A few states operate special programs for sexual offenders. In the Federal Bureau of Prisons forensic services to federal courts are often provided by the staff of the Bureau's mental health facilities.

A few mental health facilities in the corrections field seek accreditation from JCAHO. There is also a relevant set of standards specifically targeted to jails published by the National Commission on Correctional Health Care (NCCHC 1996). These standards may also be helpful in the design and operation of programs.

Administrative problems in corrections programs may be unique. Jails and prisons must exercise responsibility for public safety as a primary objective and thus security is an ever-present administrative problem. Control of violence, even to staff, is always an issue. In prisons there is a paucity of resources and clinical personnel. Physical facilities emphasize security rather than a therapeutic environment. There appears to be a high degree of treatment resistance, chronicity, and chemical abuse comorbidity that distinguishes the prison populations' mentally ill. In jails there are similar problems with security, a limitation of resources, a high suicide risk, and too few diversion programs for the less serious offender. Relationships between corrections and mental health authorities may be complicated by divergence in philosophies between the two.

Managed Care Organizations

Managed care organizations (MCOs) assume many different forms and are growing and evolving rapidly in the United States. Indeed, Stroup and

Dorwart (1997) state as follows: "Cataclysmic changes taking place in the name of 'managed care' threaten the very foundations of public sector mental health care."

But it is not only the public sector in which managed care is growing. Mental health services in the private sector are being managed by organizations. More than 120 million persons now have managed behavioral health care insurance coverage (Manderscheid and Henderson 1996). Mechanic (1996) refers to hundreds of organizations that are involved in the management of mental health services although a few large organizations dominate the field.

In fact, managed care is not a single type of organization but a variety of organizations including Health Maintenance Organizations (HMOs), Behavioral Health Care Corporations (BHCCs), Utilization Management (UM) organizations, Preferred Provider Organizations (PPOs), and subvariations within all the categories.

Among HMOs there is great variability. At least four major variants exist (Mechanic 1996). These are briefly described as follows:

Group Model HMO. Services are provided under contract with a plan on a capitated basis by a multi-specialty group.

Staff Model HMO. The services are provided by staff members hired by the HMO, which is a capitated organization.

Network Model. The HMO contracts with a number of groups of providers who provide care for the patients at a capitated rate.

Independent Practice Associations (IPA). Practitioners affiliate and form an HMO that contracts on a capitation basis but provides services in each individual's office. Such providers usually do not limit care to HMO members but may provide fee-for-service care and even may see patients from other HMOs. This category of HMO is growing rapidly.

Other managed care organizations exist besides HMOs. PPOs are plans in which the insurance organization contracts with providers at reduced rates. Point of Service (POS) plans provide enrollees access to providers outside the plan, but usually require additional copayment. Some HMOs also include an option for POS, again with increased fees or copayments to the enrollee. UM organizations typically do not provide direct services but oversee the utilization of services for a payer using techniques such as pre-certification and concurrent review. Some even require the use of approved treatment protocols or the establishment of a clear treatment plan with goals and objectives. Managed care may also include employee assistance programs, health education, and illness prevention programs.

In addition to these variations, the financing plans are highly variable, ranging from full capitation to partial capitation from no-risk to full-risk. Provider fees may be discounted by PPOs. Some HMOs employ incentive devices such as risk pools, which used to be used as performance bonuses, and withholding, in which partial withholding of the capitation payment is made but is returned to the provider upon meeting of financial targets.

An HMO is not obligated to provide mental health service if it is not a federally qualified HMO. But participation in Medicare or Medicaid funding requires federal qualification. The organization with which an HMO contracts can opt for a range of mental health services that it desires. Most HMOs do provide some mental health benefits. **Mainstreaming** of mental health services within the overall HMO benefit package is the most common practice but some HMOs will opt for **carve-out programs** in which mental health services are contracted out to a separate organization on either a capitated basis or a fixed-fee basis.

Carve-out is a more common method of providing services to those patients who require a high volume of mental health services, a level or type of service not generally represented within the HMO, or extensive support services. Because of the high level of service and high cost of chronically and severely mentally ill or severely emotionally disturbed children, these groups are prime candidates for carve-out programs. This is especially true for public mental health programs in which there is a high representation of both groups. The carve-out program may face problems in the provision of basic health services for which it often does not have the facilities or personnel. As a result, it must have elaborate referral and coordination mechanisms with the HMO or, in turn, subcontract for basic health services.

Physician participation in HMOs is much higher for the medical and surgical specialties than it is for psychiatrists although some HMOs have multi-disciplinary mental health teams as part of their staff or group.

MCOs can be expected to meet standards for accreditation. Managed Behavioral Healthcare Organizations (MBHOs) will be expected to meet specific standards to achieve accreditation. Among the various standards, the most specific set is Standards for Accreditation of Managed Behavioral Healthcare Organizations (NCQA 1977). Administrators can also use these standards to assist them in service delivery design and quality evaluation. These standards place much emphasis on member satisfaction.

The administrative issues involved in managed behavioral health care

are potentially enormous and include cost accounting, competitive cost analysis, methods of capitation, management of at-risk and risk-sharing contracts, internal utilization review, integrated financial and clinical management systems, billing capabilities and quality assurance, and improvement. Besides these, the system must provide for a range of appropriate clinical services including twenty-four-hour emergency intake and triage, inpatient care and/or hospital diversion programs, outpatient services, medication management, non-hospital residential care, and any and all clinical and supportive services whether it is a mainstream or carve-out program.

Another important aspect of managed care is the emergence of managed care of Medicaid programs, especially that of managing mental health services. Medicaid along with Medicare are the greatest source of funds for public mental health services. Beginning in 1991, states began to obtain the necessary Medicaid waivers and to develop management strategies for the expenditure of Medicaid funds. **Almost all states have initiated such managed care strategies or have applied for the necessary waivers.**

The pattern of managed public mental health Medicaid expenditures is very diverse. No two states appear to be alike. For example, Tennessee and Massachusetts elected to begin with mainstreaming while Iowa, Oregon, and Utah developed carve-out programs. Frank, McGuire, Notman, and Woodward describe the following approaches to managed care by the states:

> 1) inclusion of behavioral health as part of benefits included in capitated HMO arrangements, 2) statewide carve-out programs where behavioral health services are managed separately from other care, 3) specialty carve-outs where only care for persons with severe mental illness (SMI) or other high risk groups are managed separately, and 4) mixed approaches of carve-out and HMO arrangements. (Frank et al. 1996:138)

A unique problem being faced by the states is the significant numbers of high-risk patients, either adults with serious mental illness or children who are seriously emotionally disturbed. If an HMO approach is used, the capitation rate must be adjusted to account for the risk of such patients. Carve-out programs must adjust rates to account for the risk characteristics of the population served.

Some states have contracted with private MCOs to administer the program while others have solicited new MCOs from existing service entities. Most state managed care services, however, rely heavily on community mental health programs to serve as providers, especially to high-risk patients.

The administration of managed Medicaid / mental health programs is complex. The programs generally deal with a large number of provider groups in many and diverse locations. All the administrative issues discussed here apply to these programs. In addition, the large numbers of high-risk patients require special capitation rates and require the availability of many support and collateral services.

Miscellaneous Mental Health Organizations

In addition to the major delivery systems described here, there remains a diverse and heterogeneous group of organizations that provide mental health services. Examples include school counseling programs, mental health services in universities, academically based treatment programs, Indian Health Service or tribal mental health services, marriage and family services, rehabilitation programs, and pastoral counseling. Each has its own unique characteristics.

GLOSSARY

Accreditation A determination that an organization meets the standards established by the accrediting agency such as JCAHO, CARF, or NCQA

BHCC A Behavioral Health Care Corporation is a corporate entity specializing in the delivery of behavioral health care services

BHO A Behavioral Health Care Organization is an organization specializing in the delivery of behavioral health care services

CARF The Commission on Accreditation of Rehabilitation Facilities is a national not-for-profit organization which establishes standards for and accredits organizations serving people with disabilities

Carve-out The process of segregating a portion of a population for purposes of providing medical and health services through an organization different from the customary HMO services delivery system

CHAMPUS The Civilian Health and Medical Program for the Uniformed Services which provides medical and health care to the dependents of military service personnel through contractual arrangements with private practitioners and organizations

Comorbidity The existence of a second disease process in conjunction with the primary disease process

Federal qualification Federal qualification refers to the approval of an HMO to provide services to Medicare patients

HMO A Health Maintenance Organization which provides medical and health services under contract to a general population under a capitated payment plan

IPA An Independent Practice Association is an organization of practitioners to form an HMO in which services are delivered in the practitioners' own offices

JCAHO The Joint Commission on Accreditation of Healthcare Organizations is a national not-for-profit organization which sets standards for and accredits a variety of organizations which deliver health care services and was formerly known as the Joint Commission on Accreditation of Hospitals

Mainstreaming The inclusion of a special population into the customary HMO services delivery system

MBHCO A Managed Behavioral Health Care Organization which contracts to deliver behavioral health care services to a specific population under a capitated payment plan

MCO A Managed Care Organization which contracts to provide health services to a specific population in a specific manner which may be an HMO, a PPO, or an IPA.

Medicare certification The determination by the Health Care Financing Administration (HCFA) that a hospital meets the conditions required by the administration's rules and regulations, thereby qualifying the hospital to be reimbursed for the care of Medicare patients

Medicaid 1915B waiver An authorization by the Health Care Financing Administration for a state Medicaid plan to modify the requirement that Medicaid services be available uniformly in the state, thus allowing flexibility such as implementing managed care in some areas or for some population

Medicaid 1115 waiver An authorization for a state Medicaid plan to accomplish all allowed under a 1915B waiver but also to extend eligibility to other populations and to use HMO and PPO model programs

NAPHS The National Association of Psychiatric Health Systems, formerly known as NAPPH (National Association of Private Psychiatric Hospitals)

NASMHPD The National Association of State Mental Health Program Directors is an organization representing the SMHAs at a national level

NCQA The National Committee for Quality Assurance is a national not-for-profit organization that sets standards for and accreditations managed care organizations

POS A Point of Service Plan is one that allows for the delivery of services by providers who are not part of the HMO or PPO but generally with additional cost to the recipient of services

PPO A Preferred Provider Organization is an entity that contracts to provide medical and health services to a population through specific providers with which it generally contracts for such services at established reduced rates of payment

Provider panel A listing of those providers of medical and health services authorized to provide services to the beneficiaries of an HMO, PPO, IPA, or insurance plan

Risk pool The creation of a pool of monies by a Managed Care Organization (MCO) that is used at the end of a contract period to reward providers for achievement of performance standards established by the MCO

Scatter beds Those general medical or surgical beds of a hospital to which mental health patients may be admitted but which are not dedicated or reserved for such patients

SMHA A State Mental Health Authority is the agency of the state government authorized to administer that state's mental health program

UM Utilization management is the process of reviewing and controlling health care service usage through such means as preauthorization and concurrent review. An organization that specializes in such a service is a UM organization or corporation

Withholding The withholding of a pool of monies from the capitation payment by an MCO to providers until such time as the providers meet the performance standards established by the MCO

REFERENCES

Commission on Accreditation of Rehabilitation Facilities (CARF). 1998. *Standards Manual for Organizations Serving People with Disabilities.* Tucson, AZ: Commission on Accreditation of Rehabilitation Facilities.

Community Mental Health Centers Act (CMHC). 1963. P.L. 88–164.

DuRand, C. J., G. J. Burtka, E. J. Federman, J. A. Haycox, and J. W. Smith. 1995. A Quarter Century of Suicide in a Major Urban Jail: Implications for Community Psychiatry. *American Journal of Psychiatry* 152 (7): 1077.

Frank, R. E., T. G. McGuire, E. H. Notman, and R. M. Woodward. 1996. Developments in Medicaid Managed Behavioral Health Care. In R. W. Mansfield and M. A. Sonnerschein, eds., *Mental Health, United States, 1996.* Rockville, MD: Center for Mental Health Services, Substance Abuse and Mental Health Administration, U.S. Department of Health and Human Services.

Joint Commission on Accreditation of Healthcare Organizations (JCAHO). 1999. *Behavioral Health Care Manual, 1999–2000.* Oakbrook Terrace, IL: Joint Commission on Accreditation of Healthcare Organizations.

Joint Commission on Accreditation of Healthcare Organizations (JCAHO). 1998. *Comprehensive Accreditation Manual for Hospitals, 1998.* Oakbrook Terrace, IL: Joint Commission on Accreditation of Healthcare Organizations.

Lamb, H. R. and L. E. Weinberger. 1998. Persons with severe mental illness in jails and prisons: A review. *Psychiatric Services* 49 (4): 483–92.

Manderscheid, R. W. and M. J. Henderson. 1996. The Growth and Direction of Managed Care. In R. W. Mansfield and M. A. Sonnerschein, eds., *Mental Health, United States, 1996.* Rockville, MD: Center for Mental Health Services, Substance Abuse and Mental Health Administration, U.S. Department of Health and Human Services.

Mechanic, D. S. 1996. Key Policy Decisions for Mental Health in the Managed Care Era. In R. W. Mansfield and M. A. Sonnerschein, eds., *Mental Health, United States, 1996.* Rockville, MD: Center for Mental Health Services, Substance Abuse and Mental Health Administration, U.S. Department of Health and Human Services.

National Association of Psychiatric Health Systems (NAPHS). 1997. *Annual Survey Report.* Washington, DC: National Association of Psychiatric Health Systems.

National Association of State Mental Health Program Directors (NASMHPD). 1996. *FY96 SMHA Profiling System, Narrative Highlights.* Alexandria, VA: National Association of State Mental Health Program Directors.

National Commission on Correctional Health Care (NCCHC). 1996. *Standards for Health Services in Jails.* Chicago: National Commission on Correctional Health Care.

National Committee for Quality Assurance (NCQA). 1997. *Standards for the Accreditation of Managed Behavioral Healthcare Organizations.* Washington, DC: National Committee for Quality Assurance.

Redick, R. W., M. J. Witkin, J. A. Atay, and R. W. Manderscheid. 1996. Highlights of Organized Mental Health Services in 1997 and Major National and State Trends. In R. W. Mansfield and M. A. Sonnerschein, eds., *Mental Health, United States, 1996.* Rockville, MD: Center for Mental Health Services, Substance Abuse and Mental Health Administration, U.S. Department of Health and Human Services.

Rowen, J. R., and L. M. Hayes. 1995. *Training Curriculum on Suicide Detection and Treatment in Jails and Lockups,* 2d ed. Washington, DC: National Center on Institutions and Alternatives, U.S. Department of Justice.

Stroup, T. S., and R. A. Dorwart. 1977. Overview of Public Sector Managed Mental Health Care. In K. Minkoff and D. Pollack, eds., *Managed Mental Health Care in the Public Sector: A Survival Manual.* Amsterdam: Harwood Academic Publishers.

CHAPTER 3

Marketing Mental Health Services

E. Gordon Whyte, Ph.D., and William F. Martin, Psy.D., M.P.H., M.A.

Practitioners are beginning to hear a different language being spoken in the halls and conference rooms of most mental health organizations. This language is the language of marketing and sales. Mental health administrators and practitioners are used to discussing needs assessments and catchment areas. Yet it has only been in recent times that administrators and practitioners are talking about market research, niche markets, segmentation, and forecasting. This change in language reflects the change in the organization, financing, and delivery of all types of health care including mental health care.

Changes in the health care delivery system are impacting the way in which services are delivered and the way that patients learn about them. Patients are growing into a well-informed group of consumers who not only want choices but also want information on which to base their choices.

In fact, *choice* may be the operative word in successful delivery of health care services at the millennium. There is a transition going on right now that is based on the shifting tides in the marketplace between cost saving/cutting and choice. As managed care organizations and plans have grown over the last ten years, individuals and organizations have seen their options in accessing health care services become more limited for the sake of and in the name of cost savings and efficiency.

Conservative cost-minded individuals and companies, who in the past were critics of the medical care system, have adopted the rhetoric of corporate America in this debate between cost and choice. What was once feared as the socialization of medicine is now heralded as the new corporate form of medicine (Starr 1982).

Many people believe that one of the inherent characteristics of being American is a desire for choice in our lives. We have always wanted to be free to choose our schools, our homes, our cars, our churches. We have fought political and social battles to ensure that we have the final word in all of these and other things that impact our daily lives. We also took for granted the choice we had about which doctor to see and when to see the doctor. That was until the successful integration of managed care programs into the system.

The idea of managed care is not a new one. In fact, the concept of prepayment for a package of health care services can be traced back to the early 1900s in the Pacific Northwest where lumber, mining, and transportation companies sought to compensate for the unavailability of suitable health care for their employees by hiring their own doctors (Starr 1982). In the 1970s the federal government entered the debate on the side of managed care by way of the adoption of the Nixon Health Care Policy and the passage of the HMO Act of 1973 (PL 93-222). In the 1990s business weighed in again, this time not seeking to improve access to health care services but rather seeking relief from escalating costs of available services.

At that point, the concept of cost-benefit, familiar to business in many other circumstances, began to be applied to purchase of health benefits. With the cost-benefit application to health services by business, the importance of the purchasers of health benefits took on new meaning for the providers in the health care industry. Prior to this time, most attention was given to the providers of services and their needs and demands, followed by attention to the users (patients) and their needs and demands. Now the attention has been focused on the purchasers, usually businesses and, of course, the federal government.

Today's managed care plans are introducing more point of service (POS) type of options that allow the patients more choice in the selection of the providers of their health care. Choice is not just essential in the selection of health services but plays a role in every selection of every product and service that a consumer makes.

Consumer behavior is a heavily researched and understood set of processes. It remains at times, however, unpredictable. Marketing is the ability of an organization to identify its consumers, to offer products and services that are designed to meet the needs, wants, and demands of those consumers, while ensuring that the consumers know what services and products are being offered and why the organization's particular services and products best meet their needs, wants, and demands.

Thus the marketplace is filled with consumers needing, wanting, and demanding more choice and "say-so" in their health care. Simultaneously, the health care providers are faced with greater pressures from the purchasers to deliver health care services more efficiently (low cost) and effectively (successful outcomes) and compassionately (service excellence).

Additionally, provider organizations are faced with not only more competition from traditional health care providers but also with a growing interest in nontraditional providers of service that expand the number and scope of the competitors for the consumers' interest.

These consumer and competitive pressures combine to necessitate the use of marketing for the development of services, and the positioning of health care organizations in the marketplace. **Marketing has become critical to the survival and prosperity of any health care organization. Mental health organizations are no exception.**

The marketing function can take many different forms within mental health organizations. These forms can include a distinct marketing department, a dedicated marketing staff, a single marketing professional, and a marketing budget and process. No matter which form the marketing activities take, the key to success is the adoption of a true marketing orientation throughout the entire organization. As defined by Kotler:

> A marketing orientation holds that the main task of the organization is to determine the needs and wants of target markets and to satisfy them through the design, communication, pricing, and delivery of appropriate and competitively viable products and services. (1997:31)

There are other orientations to marketing. Some of them are more prevalent in health care organizations. Payne (1988) and Levitt (1960) describe three such orientations. They are a production orientation, product orientation, and sales orientation. In fact, health care organizations today tend to gravitate to a production orientation in those markets that have significant managed care penetration rates. A production orientation focuses on cost reductions and gains in efficiency in the production of the services. Good examples of the production orientation are companies that pride themselves on the smooth flow of patients through the system without sensitivity to the individual needs of each patient on each day. Physicians sometimes have patients wait long periods of time so that they may work efficiently.

Many behavioral health care organizations reflect a product orientation. Product oriented organizations are in love with their product. They violate the old marketing axiom "love the customer, not the product." Implicit in this orientation to health services is the attitude that "we know what you need more than you do," unfortunately still found in some behavioral health organizations. According to Kotler, "the product orientation is a paternalistic approach to marketing" (1987:29). Product orientation also subtly encourages the provider to ignore patient satisfaction because the provider "knows that they provide a high quality service."

Mental health care organizations that are in highly competitive managed care markets or markets where integrated delivery systems are the prime providers frequently find themselves adopting a sales orientation. A sales orientation emphasizes the maximum use of the current services through sales efforts rather than changing the services to adapt to the needs of the patients. An example in behavioral health might be selling inpatient service because there are empty beds.

No single orientation to marketing can stand alone. Efficient and effective behavioral health care organizations must adopt the right mix of the four orientations (Kotler and Clark 1987). **The closer an organization can move to the development of a marketing orientation, however, the greater the possibility that the organization will design services at the right time in the right way for the right customers.** When an organization can do this, it moves closer to the dimension that Drucker (1973) describes as the point where "marketing is so basic that it cannot be considered a separate function of management. Rather, it is the whole business seen from the point of view of the end result, that is, from the customer's point of view."

In addition to the purchasers and the consumers that have been addressed so far, marketing must also look at the needs, wants, and demands of internal customers, namely the employees of the provider organization. By extension, the employees of a purchaser organization are also internal customers of the purchaser's Employee Assistance Program (EAP). So, **there are three customer groups in the marketplace that behavioral health care organizations must address in their marketing planning: purchasers, consumers, and internal customers.**

The role of marketing, then, is to ensure that everything that everyone in the organizations does is guided by the needs, wants, and demands of the various purchasers, consumers, and internal customers. The role of the marketing function in the organization is to influence the use of the organization's services by these groups in such ways that the organization survives and prospers through the accomplishment of its mission, goals, and objectives. The first step in the process is to know more about the market and the three customer groups.

Marketing Information and Research

A chasm exists between the providers of behavioral health services and the purchasers and consumers of their services. The wider the chasm the greater the chance for poor service, poor quality, poor performance, reduced choices, and poor customer satisfaction. The aim of effective marketing is to narrow this chasm. The chasm narrowing process begins with the collection of valid and reliable information that informs the executives and managers about the needs, preferences, and wants of both purchasers and consumers of existing services and needed services yet to be developed.

The collection of data that will be converted into usable marketing information is most effectively done through the development and implementation of a marketing information system (MrkIS).

Like any other information system in the organization, **the MrkIS is designed to gather, analyze, synthesize, store, and disseminate information that is relevant and important to those people involved in marketing planning and implementation in the organizations.**

The Internal Information System

The MrkIS collects data from any number of sources. There is a wealth of information already collected by any behavioral health organization that is critical to the development of a successful MrkIS. This information is found in the internal records of the organization.

All behavioral health care organizations collect and store information on their current and past patients. When this information is being collected it is generally not for the purposes of marketing services in the future. But this information, when reviewed from a marketing perspective, contains valuable information about the current and past *customers* of the organization. This is where marketing information gathering starts. **The organization must come to a thorough understanding of who their current customers are and analyze what they need, want, and demand from the organization.**

The risk of violating any patient confidentiality is minimal because the marketing function is not interested in the identity of any individual patient. Rather, it is important to come to know the current patients as a group of consumers. From these internal records, the organization can develop a profile or profiles of groups of patients, their demographics, their usage patterns, their charges and costs, their referral sources, and other useful information. Once an organization begins to see the internal records as marketing information sources, improvements in the type of information collected, and the efficiency and effectiveness of collecting the information are easily identified and implemented. As anyone who has delved into the development of information systems recently can testify, this can become not only an overwhelming task but a very expensive one too. **The goal of the development of the MrkIS is not to develop the most**

expensive and comprehensive system but rather to develop the most useful and relevant one in terms of the intended use of the information by those charged with marketing the organization and its services.

The best way to begin this process is through discussions with the employees who are charged with marketing the organization. What is it that they need to know and in what form would it be most useful to them? Develop a list of questions that the system will be designed to answer.

Good MrkISs are user-friendly but technology-dependent. It is no longer feasible to think that an organization can compile data and manage it into useful information without the aid of computers. Even with the use of technology, adequate time must be allowed for the collection and input of the data into the system. This step is important and time-consuming. But the information is only as good as the data on which it is constructed. There are packaged MrkISs available. They are most useful and most economical if they can be used without modification. Otherwise, it is likely that the development of a unique internal system will be more economical, and its specific design will better meet the needs of the particular organization.

The External Information System

The collection, analysis, synthesis, and dissemination of external marketing information is called marketing research. There are basically three ways of doing marketing research: do it yourself, hire someone to do it for you, or purchase the information from an outside source.

Organizations with in-house marketing staffs may have the capability and talent to produce high quality marketing research themselves. Yet, like any type of scientific research, if done correctly, this effort will be time consuming and expensive.

There are several ways to go about gathering the information, each requiring careful planning and execution. The most common methods include survey research and focus group research.

Survey research is undertaken to identify, first hand, the magnitude and strength of selected market segments attitudes, preferences, knowledge, and beliefs about the organization, its services, and those of the competition. Marketing surveys are conducted in several different ways. One of the more common ways is the marketing telephone survey. In doing telephone marketing research, careful thought has to be given to the objectives of the study and the wording of questions. The order and sequencing of the questions as well as their construction is very important. Just as important to the successes of the method is the training of the surveyors.

These individuals must be able to garner enough interest from the responders to not only keep them on the line but also get them to honestly answer the questions without hostility or prejudice. **A professional telephone marketing firm is recommended to ensure thoroughness, completeness, and professionalism of the interviews.**

A second survey technique used in marketing research is the written survey. Like written surveys of all kinds, there must be some reason for the respondent to participate, an incentive. The incentive can range anywhere from a token that arrives with the survey, to a coupon for some gift or service for the completed questionnaire. The written survey is frequently used in patient satisfaction surveys. Health care organizations rarely offer any type of incentive for responses, however, and therefore response rates are typically low.

While mall intercept interviews are not typically used by health care organizations, they are one of the more popular survey methods used for consumer products and could have some usefulness if the behavioral health organizations are going to target populations that frequent malls such as teenagers or healthy mobile elderly.

The focus group has grown in popularity in recent years, in health care and in many other industries as well. A focus group is a group of eight to twelve individuals carefully screened and selected to represent a particular demographic, or characteristic that is felt by the health care organization to be important and relevant to the success of a particular service or product. The group is recruited and brought together at an assigned time and place to discuss certain ideas, services, organizational image, or any specified topic that lends itself to group discussion. The group members are usually paid a fee for their participation, generally somewhere between twenty-five and fifty dollars. Refreshments are generally served during the group discussion. The group leader should be a professionally trained discussion leader who has experience in ferreting out opinions from individuals in a group setting and who can bring the group to some sort of consensus about the subject of the focus group. **In an effort to avoid surveyor bias in the facilitation of the group discussion, it is usually not recommended that a member of the host organization conduct the group.**

Focus group research is not generalizable. It is not intended to generate information that is necessarily true for the rest of the target population. Remember that the sample in a focus group is very small and is never random. Information gathered from focus group sessions should be considered like a pilot test of a new idea or service concept. **It would be extremely risky to go to market with ideas and/or services that only have been researched through focus groups.**

The Characteristics of Good Marketing Research

Without good research to back up its marketing plans, an organization is acting on little more than the intuition and instinct of its managers. While these attributes have a role to play in marketing decision making, they should not be allowed to dominate the process. Kotler (1997) has clarified seven characteristics of good marketing research that can guide managers in the development of a research plan and in the selection of a research firm.

First, good marketing research uses the principles of scientific method, that is, careful observation, formulation of hypotheses, prediction, and finally testing. So, the marketer must first watch what is going on in the marketplace (observation), form some opinion about why the marketplace is acting the way it is (hypothesis), establish a list of possible solutions or activities that are thought to affect the marketplace's activities with regard to the services of the organization (prediction), and then test the predictions through research methods intended to give insight into the possible success of the predictions (testing).

Second, research has to be creative. Each step of the process allows for the researchers to pose creative observations, hypotheses, and predictions. Good researchers will also have the ability to find innovative ways of collecting information. They are not limited to the few techniques or approaches generally accepted as "marketing research." A major part of successful marketing is creativity and it begins in the research process.

Third, don't be afraid to use multiple methods. Particularly, beware of always using the same method no matter what the research objective.

Fourth, the data collected are interpreted based on the model used to construct the research. Therefore, the models should be explicitly expressed and the objective of the study clearly articulated.

Fifth, recognize that the collection and analysis of data have a cost and that the costs should be evaluated in light of the real value of the information. The difficulty usually lies in estimating the value of the information. The cost of the research is usually easily calculatable.

Sixth, in almost every organization, there is an underlying feeling that they know their markets, meaning that marketing research is unnecessary because of the good observations and intuition of management. A healthy skepticism of this assertion is needed to ensure good marketing research.

Seventh, good marketing research is done in compliance with good marketing ethics. Some individuals see marketing research as intrusive to their privacy. Additionally, the privacy of individual patient information must be protected in all cases.

The marketing research process in some circles of health care industry is better known and accepted as needs assessment. The basic tenets remain the same. It is most important that marketing research and needs assessment be framed from a holistic perspective as suggested by Jaffee (1982:386). Specifically, Jaffee posits that "the assessment of needs of the mental health center's target population should be the foundation for the planning and delivery of relevant and meaningful mental health services at the community, county, and state levels."

When Not to Do Marketing Research

There are times when the circumstances dictate that marketing research will not serve the needs of the organization, even when a marketing campaign or marketing response is called for. The first has already been mentioned, when the cost of the research will exceed the value of the research. There is also a variation on this same theme that says that marketing research should not be pursued when there simply is inadequate budget to adequately support it. Another contraindication for marketing research is when time is of the essence or when the organization is in a reactive situation brought on by the aggressive move of a competitor. **Thorough marketing research cannot be done on the fly. It takes time to develop the objective, the instruments, and the approaches.** It is worth mentioning, however, that a well-developed marketing information system can reduce the possibilities that the competition can make such a surprise move.

Just as an organization should not rush the research process because it will not have time to adequately develop the entire process, it should not pursue marketing research without clear goals and specific objectives for the project. Nonspecific marketing research will provide nonspecific marketing information. This approach turns the research into the same kind of guessing game that nonresearched marketing campaigns often result in. Save your money if you don't know what you are looking for.

Another instance where an organization might not want to invest in research is when it is known that the research will not represent the future of the marketplace. If sweeping change is about to be introduced into the marketplace, it might be more beneficial to allow the change to begin and the marketplace to respond before measuring particular positions, attitudes, and other attributes.

Finally, **an organization should not invest its time, effort, and financial resources in collecting data and information that already exist. Take advantage of others' work particularly if you know it to be credible.**

Deciding to Do Marketing Research

Before deciding to implement a marketing research effort, the following ten question should all be answered:

1. What will be accomplished through the marketing research project?
2. What questions are we going to ask that the research project will answer?
3. What information is going to be needed?
4. Is the information already available within the organization?
5. Is the information already available outside of the organization?
6. How will the information be analyzed? And by whom?
7. What market area is important to cover in the research?
8. What are the time constraints on the research project?
9. What will the research project cost?
10. How valuable will the information really be?

Forecasting, Segmenting, and Targeting the Behavioral Health Market

Forecasting

Today's behavioral health services environment is radically different from what it was ten years ago. These differences have not only impacted the way that mental health organizations do business but they have also changed the way that mental health professionals provide services.

The successful mental health organization or practitioner must adopt the marketing orientation discussed earlier in order to participate in the managed care sector of the marketplace. Why? According to Winegar and Bistline (1994:34) there are three compelling reasons: (1) managed care systems will not automatically include all practitioners in the community; (2) managed care systems will refer to clinicians and organizations that can provide the services valued by the system's members; (3) the decision concerning the credentialing of practitioners or organizations (the purchasing decision) is made by health care managers, not by the lay public.

Today's clinicians have to develop practice styles that are compatible with the demands of the marketplace including managed care, alternative medicine, strong competition as a result of more available practitioners, and the continuing misunderstanding of the role and benefits of mental health services in a community.

Because of this shift in the marketplace and the resultant changes in mental health organization and practitioners, the ability to accurately forecast demand has become more important. The market forecast shows the expected level of market demand for an organization's services in a given market environment. If the environment changes then the demand would be expected to change as well. Therefore, the organization should carefully define the characteristics of the marketing environment before starting to forecast the demand for the services.

The expected level of market demand for mental health services in a given environment can be forecast by adjusting Kotler's (1997) formula for total market potential. Thus, the adjusted formula for forecasting demand for mental health services is:

$$MD = nbqd$$

where: MD = market demand; n = total number of people that could use mental health services in a given period of time; b = number of people likely to use mental health services in the same time period; q = the level (or number) of services that a typical person seeking services will use in the given time period; d = dollars allowed (reimbursed) per typical course of treatment in the marketplace.

Segmenting

Both internal and external marketing information will be necessary in order to understand who the current customers are and who the future customer can be. Because of the increasing trend of specialization among behavioral health providers, the identification of existing referral sources and the development of marketing strategies are key activities (Gevirtz 1990).

When collecting the internal and external marketing information, identifiable groups of patients will be revealed. Additionally, other groups of patients or potential patients can be created from the information about the marketplace. These groups are referred to by marketers as segments.

The study of consumer behavior represents one of the cornerstones of marketing and sales. The ultimate outcome in both the clinical and business world is to change the behavior of individuals and groups in a desired direction. Clinical practitioners design and implement treatment plans to modify patient behavior and eventually improve patient functioning, as measured by changes in specific behaviors, for example, phobic behaviors. Marketing and sales professionals develop and implement marketing and sales campaigns to modify the purchasing decisions and consumption behaviors of a specific target market, for instance, a "Fear of Flying" clinic.

The science of segmenting a market falls into two broad domains: demographics and psychographics. The demographic approach to segmentation presumes that individual consumers make purchasing decisions and engage in discrete consumer behaviors based upon some identifiable demographic characteristics. For instance, patients under the age of 30 and those that have earned a degree in one of the technical sciences might be more likely to respond to an advertisement for mental health services on the World Wide Web.

The psychographic approach to market segmentation presumes that individual consumers are better segmented based upon both their view of the world and the behavioral style that characterizes their purchasing decisions. Psychographics are psychological profiles that break down the marketplace into segments based on lifestyles, personality characteristics, or buying motives and that identify specific purchasing behaviors of the identified segments. For example, a "Fear of Public Speaking" workshop might attract two distinct types of buyers—one set will attempt to determine the cost-benefit ratio and attend only if the benefits outweigh the costs; another set will see the advertisement, respond impulsively, and attend.

Clinical practitioners and mental health organizations should identify the demographic and psychographic composition of their existing clientele and potential clientele. One of the more effective and efficient ways to assess the composition of your current clientele is to include in the MrkIS, a computerized database, a process that will allow you to search on key demographic characteristics as well as write reports soliciting particular information. For example, what is the distribution of my clientele that speaks Spanish? If you discover that 20 percent of your clientele speaks Spanish, then you can identify the types of services that this population might find attractive. It is critical that you realize that demographic characteristics represent a moving target. For instance, the percentage of your clientele that speaks Spanish may be only 20 percent today, but it could conceivably be 50 percent within a five-year period. Are you prepared for a 250 percent jump in the percentage of clientele that speaks Spanish?

The identification of demographic characteristics is easier than psychographic characteristics. In-depth individual interviews and focus group interviews represent two tools that will assist you, however, in identifying specific psychological characteristics that have an impact on purchasing decisions and behaviors. Individuals that have suffered a heart attack, a stroke, or any other life-threatening cardiovascular or cerebrovascular event are often very motivated to modify their lifestyle with respect to exercise, nutrition, and stress management. Why?—the life-threatening event set of a cascade of emotional, behavioral, and cognitive dynamics that forced the individuals to break through denial and reach out for professional assistance. What can an individual clinical practitioner or mental health organization do with this information? The answer is simple. Develop a promotional strategy (that will be discussed later in this chapter) to increase awareness among these patients, their families, cardiologists, neurologists, cardiac rehabilitation centers, and discharge planners about you as an expert, your organization, and the tailored services provided for patients who have suffered life-threatening events.

Targeting

Deciding which segments of the marketplace to serve is one of the most important and strategic marketing decisions. Once a segment or multiple segments is selected, all future marketing decisions revolve around the individual needs, wants, and demands of the targeted segments. Marketing strategies range from a mass marketing strategy, providing all services for all segments, to a niche strategy, selecting a small number of segments, sometimes only one segment, as the focus of the marketing efforts.

Mental health organizations today are tending more toward niche marketing than the mass marketing strategies of the 1970s and 1980s when mental health centers, public and private, attempted to be comprehensive, that is, all things for all people in the community.

Good targeting decisions are based on good marketing research and specifically an analysis of the current marketing situation. **The components of a simple marketplace analysis are: estimating the demand for the services; clearly dividing the market into logical and useful segments; identifying the competitor; describing the services currently offered in the marketplace by the competition and the patterns of usage of those services by the consumers.** This marketplace analysis is considered in light of the services, market share, and capabilities of your own organization.

Understanding Demand

Demand, for marketing purposes, is generally divided into two categories. Primary demand is the demand expressed by a consumer, group of consumers, or industrial and business consumers for a product or service category. This would be equivalent to getting people in the health care marketplace to demand mental health services. Selective demand is the demand expressed by these same groups for a particular brand within the category. This would be the equivalent to getting these consumers to demand mental health services from a specific clinic or practitioner.

Mental health service providers in today's marketplace face the need to generate both kinds of demands. Depending on the penetration of the marketplace by managed care companies, it is important to ensure that purchasers, usually employers, are demanding mental health coverage in their benefits packages. Having successfully created primary demand for mental health services, providers have to then generate selective demand for their services.

These different kinds of demand call for different marketing strategies and approaches. Primary demand is frequently generated by the creation of awareness of the benefits of mental health services to the employer. This calls for a strong sales function. Sales sometimes take the form of education in health care services. It also requires providers to know the needs of the purchasers and to design services and packages of services that meet those needs. This is what marketers traditionally call "product development." It is important to recognize here that the needs of the purchasers are not necessarily the same or even closely aligned with the needs of the end users.

Selective demand is generated by creating two things: brand awareness and organizational image. Brand awareness means that the purchaser and the potential user of your services are aware of you, if you are an independent practitioner, or your organization, and would consider using your services if they need mental health services.

Organizational and product/service image are critically important to successful selective demand strategies. People make purchasing decisions, including health care purchasing decisions, based on impressions and interpretations of what they believe products and service to be. Specifically, according to Levy (1985), image about a particular product or service is drawn from many sources but always includes such ideas as: knowledge about technical aspects of the product or service; awareness of other less objective (more subjective) characteristics of the product or service; their belief about the value of the product or service; and their subjective judgments about the suitability of the product or service to meet their particular need.

Using the Marketing Mix in Positioning the Organization

The weapons that marketers have available to them for positioning the organization, and its products/services in the marketplace are called the marketing mix. They are traditionally described as the "four *P*s" of marketing: product, place, price, and promotion.

The development of the right marketing mix for a given service is not a simple task. The variables within each of the four *P*s are numerous and challenging. The answers to the following five questions, however, will give the person making the marketing decisions clear indications as to where to begin: (1) Is the target market for the services? (2) Who will influence the purchasing decision? (3) What is important to these influencers? (4) Who will make the final purchase decision? (5) What is important to them?

Let's look at the components of the marketing mix and their role in the marketing strategy. The first weapon in the marketer's armamentarium is the product mix. In mental health, as in most health care, we are offering services, not tangible products. Thus, we refer to this *P* as the service mix. The service mix includes all aspects of the services such as which services are offered, by which type of professional, in which setting, as well as the naming of the services and the programs. The service mix decisions will make up the core of the marketing strategy. What could be more important to an organization than deciding which services it is going to offer? Everything else that the organization does is done to support, improve, and promote the offered services. Selecting the right services for the needs, wants, and demands of the target market is the reason that the organization exists and at the heart of why it can succeed.

The second weapon available to marketers is the place mix. Place is also frequently referred to in the marketing literature as distribution. In health care services it is most accurately thought of as access. So, the access mix answers the question, How are our customers going to get access to our services? In the managed care market access can either be through a primary care physician (PCP) or it can be through direct self referral. The difference between the two is evident and so should be the implications for developing an access strategy for the mental health service provider. If patients cannot self-refer, the mental health providers must ensure that they are treated as equal partners in the managed care plans, along with all of the other participating specialists and sub-specialists. Failure to do so will, in all likelihood, lead to a reduction of referrals from the PCP, reduced services to the patients, and reduced revenues to the provider organizations. The perception of mental health practitioners can be greatly impacted through an aggressive pursuit of relationships with other health care providers in the system, particularly the PCPs.

There are at least two other variables to consider in analyzing patient access: time and location. Time is important to patients as well as practitioners. It is becoming more necessary in the competitive environments of health care today, for health care services to be offered at times that are convenient for the patient, not just the practitioner. Evening and weekend hours are attractive to employed individuals and parents. With regard to location, it is common today to find all kinds of health care practitioners offering services in branch offices or on location in the case of large employers. These kinds of activities make it easier for patients to get to their appointments, although it may not be more convenient for the practitioner. This type of planning is clear evidence of a marketing orientation. To say the patient needs to come to where I practice is more indicative of a production or sales orientation. Which is more likely to attract more patients?

The pricing mix is the third weapon in the marketing wars. The first piece of information that is needed before developing a pricing strategy is a measure of the elasticity of demand for mental health services in the marketplace. Elasticity of demand defines the relationship between the price and the quantity demanded of a product or service. Demand is said to be elastic when a small change in the price results in a large change in the quantity demanded. Conversely, demand is said to be inelastic when changes in price have little or no impact on the demand for the product or service. The law of demand states that consumers usually buy more products or services at low prices than at higher ones.

Because of the role of third-party payers in health care, price elasticity can be very difficult to analyze. In general, however, because of the perceived insolation provided to the patient by third party payers, demand for acute health care services tends to be more inclined toward inelasticity. On the other hand, in negotiating with managed care organizations or directly with employers, demand tends to be more elastic.

The second element to consider in developing a pricing strategy is your current prices relative to the prices of your competition. These two dimensions of price in the marketplace, elasticity and competitive relativeness, will determine the role and scope of pricing in marketing mental health services.

The fourth and final weapon in the marketers arsenal is promotion. Promotion is frequently thought of as advertising. Actually, promotion is a range of activities that are designed to communicate information about the organization and its services to the consumers and potential consumers in the marketplace. The activities include advertising, publicity, and direct sales.

The potential advantage of advertising aimed at the patient must be assessed in light of the level of managed care penetration in the marketplace and the structure of the mental health benefits in the various managed care plans. If the structure of the benefit packages tends to require the use of the PCP in a gatekeeping function, very little impact may be had from direct consumer advertising. In that particular case, personal relationships of the nature that we discussed above are more likely to produce greater service levels than will advertising. *Relationship marketing* is the term for such activities, but these same activities have also been called *networking* and *direct selling*.

Publicity is achieved by placing significant news about an organization in a published medium or obtaining favorable coverage on the radio or television that is not paid for. Because publicity is not paid for by the organization, it has higher credibility than paid advertising. It is generally perceived to be more objective than advertising that is conceived, developed, and paid for by the sponsoring organization. There are however, some disadvantages. The organization loses control over the content, timing, and placement of any publicity. Thus, the news release that was planned for a Friday section of the paper may not appear until Saturday when readership is down. Or it may appear in the business section when the family section may have been more desirable.

The most effective way to minimize these kinds of disadvantages is through good press relations or public relations. Like any type of relationship, those with the press need attention. The time to establish good press relations is not when you need coverage but rather when you do not need coverage. Let the press get to know you and your organization when you are not asking them for favorable coverage of an event or the introduction of a new service. This will increase the likelihood of favorable and timely coverage when you do need it. Remember, in some cases, they are looking for stories to cover because they have regular deadlines to meet. Providing them with useful information can make their job easier and can aid the development of a mutually beneficial relationship. Furthermore, such good relations can also help should you or the organization be faced with a public relations problem.

Direct selling is used when personal attention is needed for the introduction and presentation of your services. It is also the best promotional method when a lot of information is to be presented about the services. There is less wasted coverage than with advertising and much more control than with publicity. Yet personal selling allows only for the presentation of information about the services to a limited number of customers in a given amount of time. Mental health organizations, like many health care organizations have been slow to adopt direct selling as one of the tools of the marketing function. For some reason direct selling has remained distasteful as a marketing tool while publicity and advertising have received favorable acceptance in most health care organizations. When organizations take this position, they limit their ability to address specific informational needs about their services that may best be met one on one through use of direct selling methods and techniques.

Promotional strategies take us back to the central existential question in life: Do I exist and are others aware of my existence? Naturally, clinical practitioners exist and consumers desiring the services and products of clinical practitioners exist, but can these two groups of individuals find one another? Promotion is that part of marketing that seeks to build a bridge between the practitioner and/or the mental health organization and the potential client and/or patient.

Consumer behavior is the foundation upon which a promotional strategy is formulated. Why? Adults over the age of fifty-five read newspapers more than adults under the age of thirty. As such, if you launch a service that assists seniors to cope more constructively with the aging process, then advertising in a newspaper would represent a wise investment. Moreover, if you really want to make yourself and your services known to the over-fifty-five population, then you would also advertise in newspapers that focus on the over-fifty-five market.

Clinical practitioners use a wide array of tools to accomplish the objectives of increasing awareness about themselves as practitioners and/or their organization as well as awareness about the services provided, particularly those where the practitioners are experts. These tools include but are not limited to the following: press releases; public speaking; volunteering to serve on community boards; teaching a course at the local college or university; appearing on the local television or radio show; and a host of other strategies.

Upon formulating your promotional strategy, the next step is to execute your promotional strategy. The execution step of promotion is dependent upon your financial resources, your creative talents, and your ability to manage relationships with others. Best results come from the expert planning and efficient implementation of a solid, well-thought-out, coordinated campaign. The use of seasoned professional advertising personnel and marketing firms can enhance the development and implementation of the promotional campaign. This, however, requires a substantial investment of resources. Sullivan and Vigilione (1990) describe the objectives of a promotional strategy for mental health organizations as follows: (1) increase awareness among public agencies, potential patients, physicians, and others; (2) establish yourself as an expert in a particular area; and (3) increase awareness of your products and services with potential clients, patients, and referral sources. Increasing awareness is the foundation of a solid promotional strategy.

Positioning the Organization

The strategy that leads an organization to strengthen its image in the marketplace is called a positioning strategy. Positioning in the marketplace begins and ends with what the market believes about the organization, its image. According to Rynne (1995), positive name equity is as important to a health care organization as financial equity.

An effective positioning strategy helps an organization to answer the question, How do we want the marketplace to perceive us? Rynne breaks the creation of a positioning strategy into three requirements: (1) differentiation, the position must set the organization apart from all other similar organizations or ones that offer the same services; (2) value, the position that is being sought must represent a quality, attribute, or characteristic that will be valued by the marketplace; (3) strength, the position must be based on a fundamental strength of the organization.

There are two dimensions that define any market position: what the marketplace currently thinks of the services of your organization and what the marketplace currently thinks of the services of the competition (i.e., what they think of you and what they think of them). A clear understanding of those dimensions will allow any organization to take advantage of their current position, take advantage of the position of the competing organizations, or change either or both.

There are three characteristics of an effective positioning strategy: (1) a crystal clear statement of what the intended position is; (2) a belief in the veracity and value of the position by the employees of the organization, from top to bottom; (3) a coordinated, consistent, and continuous campaign designed to communicate the position to the marketplace.

Summary

Marketing is not a new concept to many mental health care administrators. There exists a wide array of tools and techniques that can assist administrators in the design, implementation, and continuous improvement of an organization-wide marketing orientation. A marketing orientation represents the capacity of a mental health organization to identify the needs and wants of target markets and to satisfy them through the development of well-designed, clearly communicated, affordable, appropriate, competitive, and easy-to-use products and services.

The starting point in the establishment of an effective and efficient marketing orientation is the creation of a marketing information system (MrkIS). The MrkIS is similar to the diagnostic phase of the treatment planning process. In other words, the goal of the MrkIS is to clearly determine the target groups that the mental health organization have historically served, currently serve, and/or intend to serve. Some of the techniques employed include but are not limited to forecasting and qualitative market research strategies like focus group interviews. Marketing professionals refer to target groups as segments.

One of the more important strategic marketing decisions is to determine which segments of the marketplace to serve. Segments are generally categorized into demographic segments and psychographic segments.

Mental health administrators and practitioners are quite familiar with demographic segments in which the demographic characteristics predict individual consumer behavior, yet they have only recently begun to use psychographic characteristics to predict individual consumer behavior. Although the psychographic approach is relatively new to mental health administrators, the core competencies required to successfully predict individual behaviors governing purchases falls within the domain of competence of mental health professionals who have developed a thorough understanding of lifestyles, personality characteristics, and motives.

Targeting is necessary but not sufficient. The other side of the equation is the creation and utilization of rigorously sound market research. These two factors together result in a more valid and reliable analysis of the current marketing situation. The key characteristics of an effective yet simple marketplace analysis are as follows: estimating the demand for services; clearly diving the market into logical and useful segments; identifying the competitor; describing the services currently offered in the marketplace by the competition and the patterns of usage of those services by the consumers.

Another very important aspect of creating and launching a marketing orientation entails positioning the mental health organization and its products and services in a way that the organization achieves and sustains a competitive advantage. The positioning of the organization and its products/services is packaged in a framework known as the marketing mix. The marketing mix is associated with the four *P*s of marketing: product, place, price, and promotion.

The art of marketing involves the development of the right marketing mix for a given service. In order to determine the right mix, it is imperative that the following five questions be addressed prior to making any decisions:

1. Who is the target market for the services?
2. Who will influence the purchasing decision?
3. What is important to these influencers?
4. Who will make the final purchase decision?
5. What is important to them?

In essence, an effective marketing orientation depends upon a number of factors. Data collection, data analysis, and data interpretation are vital to identifying targets, segmenting markets, and positioning the organization and its products/services.

There is a truism in marketing that most of us are familiar with today. This truism is that "perception is reality." In marketing, that perception is called a "position." Administrators and even practitioners are responsible for the effective positioning of their organizations and products/services. Marketing is everybody's job. If you fail to market, you risk failing.

GLOSSARY

Advertising Any form of nonpersonal communication about a product and/or service that is paid for by a sponsor

Consumer behavior The reason and way that buyers act when considering, choosing, buying, and using products and/or services that they perceive will meet their needs, wants, and demands

Demographic segmentation Presumes that individual consumers make purchasing decisions and engage in discrete consumer behaviors based upon some identifiable demographic characteristics

Differentiation Bringing to the attention of the members of the target markets those aspects, attributes, characteristics, and differences that distinguish the products and/or services that the organization offers from those of competing organizations

Direct selling Used when personal attention is needed for the introduction and presentation of your services. It is also the best promotional method when a lot of information is to be presented about the services

Focus group A group of eight to twelve individuals carefully screened and selected to represent a particular demographic or characteristic that is felt by the health care organization to be important and relevant to the success of a particular service or product

Market forecast Shows the expected level of market demand for an organization's services in a given market environment. If the environment changes, then the demand would be expected to change as well

Marketing The ability of an organization to identify its consumers, to offer products and services that are designed to meet the needs, wants, and demands of those consumers, while ensuring that the consumers know what services and products are being offered and why the organization's particular services and products best meet their needs, wants, and demands

MIS A marketing information system is an established set of policies and procedures designed to continuously collect, analyze, and distribute pertinent information to guide planners and leaders in the process of making marketing decisions

Marketing mix The weapons that marketers have available to them for positioning the organization and its products/services in the marketplace. They are traditionally described as the four *P*s of marketing. They are product, place, price, and promotion. In health care marketing these four *P*s are translated into: product = service, place = access, price = charges, and promotion = promotion

Marketing orientation Holds that the main task of the organization is to determine the needs and wants of target markets and to satisfy them through the design, communication, pricing, and delivery of appropriate and competitively viable products and services

Positioning The strategy that leads an organization to strengthen its image in the marketplace and in the minds of the members of the target markets

Primary demand Is the demand expressed by a consumer, group of consumers, or industrial and business consumers for a product category

Psychographic segmentation Presumes that individual consumers are better segmented based upon their view of the world and the behavioral style that characterizes both their purchasing decisions. Psychographics are psychological profiles that break down the marketplace into segments based on lifestyles, personality characteristics, or buying motives and that identify specific purchasing behaviors of the identified segments

Publicity Placing significant news about an organization in a published medium or obtaining favorable coverage on the radio or television that is not paid for

Segmentation Identifying distinct groups of purchasers within the marketplace that might require, want, and/or demand distinct products and/or services. A marketer will use a specifically designed marketing mix to attract the members of each segment to their products and/or services

Selective demand The demand expressed by a consumer, group of consumers, or industrial and business consumers for a particular brand within the category

Targeting Deciding which segments of the marketplace to serve is one of the most important and strategic marketing decisions. Once a segment or multiple segments are selected, all future marketing decisions revolve around the individual needs, wants, and demands of the targeted segments

REFERENCES

Burns, J. 1993. Reform seen cutting marketing's role. *Modern Healthcare* 23:33–34.

Conlee, G. 1990. Using marketing as a tool for practice development. In E. A. Margeneau, ed., *The Encyclopedic Handbook of Private Practice.* New York: Gardner Press.

Drucker, P. 1973. *Management: Tasks, Responsibilities, and Practices.* New York: Harper and Row.

Duncan, W. J., P. M. Ginter, and L. E. Swayne. 1992. *Strategic Management of Health Care Organizations.* Boston: PWS Kent.

Gallegos, J. S. 1982. Planning and administering services for minority groups. In M. J. Austin and W. E. Hershey, eds., *Handbook of Mental Health Administration.* San Francisco: Jossey-Bass.

Gevirtz, R. N. 1990. Referral by specialty. In E. A. Margenau, ed., *The Encylopedic Handbook of Private Practice.* New York: Gardner Press.

Halgrimson, S. 1998. Arizona campaign honored as outstanding. *Practitioner* 11:1–6.

Jaffee, B. 1982. Assessing community's mental health needs. In M. J. Austin and W. E. Hershey, eds., *Handbook of Mental Health Administration.* San Francisco: Jossey-Bass.

Kotler, P. 1997. *Marketing Management: Analysis, Planning, Implementation and Control. Ninth Edition.* Englewood Cliffs, NJ: Prentice Hall.

Kotler, P., and R. N. Clarke. 1987. *Marketing for Health Care Organizations.* Englewood Cliffs, NJ: Prentice Hall.

Langone, J. 1997. Challenging the mainstream. *Time,* 12 May , 40–43.

Levitt, T. 1960. Marketing myopia. *Harvard Business Review* 38:45–56.

Loubeau, P. R., and R. Jantzen. 1998. The effect of managed care on hospital marketing orientation. *Journal of Healthcare Management* 43:229–39.

Payne, A. F. 1988. Developing a marketing-orientation. *Business Horizons* 31:46–53.

Resnick, R. J. 1998. And then there were none (the devolution of managed care). *Independent Practitioner* 18:68–70.

Rynne, T. 1995. *Healthcare Marketing in Transition: Practical Answers to Pressing Questions.* Chicago: Irwin Professional Publishers.

Rubenstein, A. 1998. Separation and divorce. *Independent Practitioner* 18:72–74.

Sullivan, J. C., and D. J. Vigilione. 1990. Public relations. In Margeneau, E. A., ed., *The Encyclopedic Handbook of Private Practice.* New York: Gardner Press.

Upton, R. I. 1997. Consumer driven health care marketing. *Managed Care Quarterly* 5:25–29.

Winegar, N., and J. Bistline. 1994. *Marketing Mental Health Services to Managed Care.* Binghamton, NY: Hawthorne Press.

Yavas, U., and D. J. Schemwell. 1996. Competing for patients and profit. *Journal of Health Care Marketing* 16:30–37

CHAPTER 4

Review Mechanisms and Regulatory Agencies

Raymond F. Patterson, M.D.

Essential components for effective mental health administration are a well-defined program for service delivery, assurance that the program consistently provides timely and appropriate services for the populations served, and an ongoing review process to assure the current competence of practitioners within the program and throughout the mental health system as a whole.

This chapter outlines some very basic criteria for establishing and maintaining the competence of individual practitioners, assuring compliance with local and federal regulations and laws, and understanding the specific requirements of various regulatory agencies whose function is to review system-wide parameters for particular patient/client/consumer populations. It will also review the developmental history of mental health "systems" in the United States to provide the reader a framework for understanding how regulatory standards became a necessary component of mental health administration.

In order to prepare for regulatory review, the mental health administrator must first consider a needs assessment for the populations served. This assessment may be based on a particular need (i.e., for mental health services); a particular population (i.e., children, geographic region, neighborhood, or other physical parameters for a given catchment area); specific or general governmental requirement for provisions of services based on local, state, or federal law or regulation; and/or a fiscal basis for profit generation, not-for-profit service provision, or cost containment. When the system is new or unestablished the needs assessment may be quite unclear for the initial administrator or administrative service. Conversely, administrators and managers who come into the system after it has already been in existence have to understand the pros and cons, pluses and minuses, and benefits and deficits of the existing system as well as having knowledge of the requirements or particular specifications generated by the funding sources, providers, and/or recipients of the services relative to that particular system. Specific areas for consideration include: (1) statutory or legal requirements, (2) funding sources, (3) managers of services, (4) providers of services, and (5) recipients of services which introduce the administrator to a wide range of issues and stakeholders. This chapter focuses on the regulatory review requirements for the system as a whole, its component parts, and the specific providers to achieve the stated mission and goals of the service delivery system.

Mental Health Service Delivery Systems

Historically, the need, availability, and cost of quality mental health services have been the most consistently considered parameters in the development of mental health service delivery systems. Initially, mental health service delivery in the United States was based largely on the concept of home care. In colonial America care of the mentally ill individual was a family responsibility requiring assistance of the community only if the problem became too serious for the family to handle and/or affected others outside the home. While the entire community had concerns about disruptive and/or dangerous behavior, the primary concern was the economic burden for the family. If, for example, either parent was unable to work because of the need to stay home and care for a mentally ill family member, the consequences to the family were dire. The sparse population in the seventeenth and early eighteenth centuries precluded the establishment of large institutions for the mentally ill, so unless an individual was dangerous, he/she lived at home in their community assisted for the most part by family and friends. Gerald Grob, in *The Mad among Us: A History of the Care of America's Mentally Ill* (1994), describes one seventeenth-century colonial community's attempt to manage a violently mentally ill individual as follows:

> When a colonial soldier who killed his mother was acquitted by reason of insanity, the court ordered him confined for life to a "small place" erected by his father in his home but at public expense.

This was clearly a family home-based model for mental health care.

With the growth of the colonial population in the late seventeenth century and associated increases in the number of dependent persons requiring some form of assistance, various Alm's Houses were developed which typically housed together the destitute, the elderly, the ill, and the insane or "distracted" (Grob 1994).

The first hospital in the colonies was established in Philadelphia as the Pennsylvania Hospital and provided services to the destitute, poor, and "lunatics." Another facility, the New York Hospital, was established in

1791, largely because of the success of the Pennsylvania Hospital. Similarly, it admitted both the physically ill and the insane. The first public mental hospital was established in the colony of Virginia in 1793. These were typically small hospitals; therefore, the majority of mentally ill individuals continued to remain in the care of their families within the community.

In 1818, as the country was experiencing continued population growth and industrialization, the first private asylum for the insane was established. The McLean Asylum of Charlestown, Massachusetts, stated as its mission "to serve the entire community." In reality, however, McLean and other small, privately funded asylums primarily served affluent patients because of the financial difficulties encountered in attempting to serve those without the ability to pay. These difficulties, coupled with the increasing need for services, led to the development of state asylums. Prior to the establishment of state asylums, many "lunatics" and others whose behavior was considered threatening or dangerous were housed in the local jails.

Recognition of the inappropriate placement of mentally ill individuals in local jails was a major influence on Dorthea Dix and the development of a national movement for moral and medical treatment for the mentally ill. Dorthea Dix first encountered mental illness in the East Cambridge jail in Massachusetts. Because of the inhumane conditions and unrealistic beliefs that were prevalent at the time, such as the absence of stoves because the insane "did not feel the cold" (McKown 1961), Ms. Dix began to inspect many other institutions and lodgings where the insane were housed. In 1843 she convinced the Massachusetts legislature to expand the Worcester Hospital in order to increase and improve services to the mentally ill. This was part of a national campaign to advocate for the founding of new, public mental hospitals and the expansion of existing facilities.

The growth of these large institutions was dramatic as families and others saw them as potentially providing better care than could realistically be provided at home. Similarly, the local police authorities began to view the hospitals as the solutions to some of their problems with dangerous and/or annoying mentally ill persons in the communities and in the jails. The development of federal and state mental hospitals in the mid-nineteenth century, including the Government Hospital for the Insane (currently known as St. Elizabeth's Hospital) in Washington, DC, was representative of this movement.

The Association of Medical Superintendents of American Institutions for the Insane, founded in 1844 (later to become the American Psychiatric Association), suggested a maximum capacity for any state hospital facility of 250 beds (Grob 1994) in order to maintain a staff-to-patient ratio that would allow the small psychiatric staff to maintain personal contact with patients. These asylums were typically built away from the major metropolitan areas to provide distance for recovery and effective management of the mentally ill persons as well as a respite for the local community. The increasing demand for admittance to these facilities by families, police agencies, and the community at large caused a major expansion in the census of such facilities with the average resident population in urban asylums founded before 1870 reaching 432 residents by 1875. Approximately one-third of these facilities had a census of between 500 and 1,000 residents (Grob 1994). Such overcrowding eventually led public facilities to shift their major focus from personalized care to maintaining order and safety. Over time, funding shortages led to a decrease in staffing, and reliance on more restrictive forms of patient management interventions such as seclusion, restraints, cold wet sheet packs, insulin shock, and isolation.

The development of other professional associations such as the American Psychological Association, the National Association of Social Workers, and the American Nurses Association continued the call for specifically qualified individuals to provide care and treatment for the mentally ill. However, the numbers of qualified personnel and availability of funding did not keep pace with the growing need.

In 1854 Thomas Kirkbride, in "Principles of Practice" (Freedman, Kaplan, and Sadock 1976), a report generated based on his experience at the Pennsylvania Hospital, listed a number of considerations and recommendations regarding the need for mental health facilities. These are listed as follows:

1. Insanity is a disorder of the brain to which under certain contingencies everyone is liable.
2. Properly and promptly treated in its early stages, it is about as curable as most other serious diseases.
3. In a great majority of cases, it is better and more successfully treated in well-organized institutions than at home.
4. It is humanity, economy, and expediency for every state to make ample and good provision for all its insane.
5. The best hospital—the best built, best arranged, and best managed—is always cheapest in the end, no matter for what class of the insane.
6. No ventilation that is not forced is worthy of the name and a perfect system of heating and ventilation is never to be omitted being alike sanitary, restorative, and economical.

7. No expense required to secure all that has been mentioned should be deemed misplaced or injudicious or beyond the means of any state on this continent.
8. A perfect classification is indispensable for proper treatment, but there should always be a protected connection of some kind between the different wards to secure efficient supervision and for convenient and economical management.
9. Separate hospitals for the recent and chronic insane are not to be recommended.
10. Overcrowding of hospitals for the insane is an evil of serious magnitude, subversion of good order, perfect discipline, and the greatest usefulness of these institutions and the best interest of the insane.
11. Abundant means for occupation, amusement, and all that comes under the head of moral treatment should be provided in every hospital.
12. As little restraint as possible should be used and only in the best interest of the patient. Mechanical restraint may be necessary but only as a remedy and under the direction of the chief medical officer.
13. The insane should never be kept in Alm's Houses or in penal institutions.
14. Insane criminals should not be treated in ordinary state hospitals nor in separate buildings on their grounds, but in structures specifically provided in other localities.
15. Under the control of a board of managers or trustees, the physician and superintendent should be the chief executive officer serving during good behavior with a compensation sufficient to enable him to devote his whole time to his duties. He should have the nomination of all other officers, with entire control of the medical, moral, and dietetic treatment of the patients, and the unrestricted power of appointment and discharge of all persons employed in their care; all other forms of management that have been tried, having proved failures.
16. Except for special forms of disease, for which they may be desirable, one-storied buildings, especially of a temporary character, have many disadvantages without corresponding advantages.
17. Appointments from political motives are to be especially deprecated, as a dangerous departure from that sound rule, which should govern every appointing power, of seeking the best men, irrespective of every other consideration.
18. The most efficient form of supervision of a hospital for the

> insane, to assure the best interests of the institution, the patients, and the community, is a board of trustees or managers of high personal character, having enlightened views, and with ample time to devote to frequent visits and a thorough discharge of their duties.

A number of the principles of practice as stated by Thomas Kirkbride in 1854 have influenced the development of regulatory agency practices and standards. These influences will be clear later in this chapter as specific requirements are discussed.

The expansion of state psychiatric hospitals continued over the next century. By the early 1950s, however, there were substantial changes and developments that had a major impact on mental health care and caused a shift from hospital to community-based care. One factor was the development of more effective antipsychotic, antidepressant, and mood-stabilizing medications, which began with the introduction of Thorazine in the 1950s. These medications began to replace other interventions such as electric convulsive therapy, insulin shock, cold wet sheet packs, and other physical restraints, and isolation/seclusion. Another change that influenced the more effective treatment of the mentally ill was the development in 1952 of a more consistent classification system for mental diseases and disorders, the *Diagnostic and Statistical Manual for Mental Disorders, Volume 1, First Edition* (DSM-1). The third major factor had to do with the more cost-effective provision of care for individuals in the community compared to the cost for hospitalization. While the expectation of cost effective community-based care was realistic for many individual patients, the need for acute and long-term hospitalization services continued to be a reality in all jurisdictions. Finally, the successful advocacy for treatment of the mentally ill in the least restrictive environment in conjunction with associated changes in civil commitment laws throughout the country influenced the reduction in usage of public mental hospitals.

In 1963 the federal Community Mental Health Centers Act mandated the creation of community mental health systems across the country. This movement began with financial assistance from the federal government to construct community mental health centers. The Center for Mental Health Services reports the number of state hospital beds declined from 264 beds per 100,000 in 1955 to 112 beds per 100,000 in 1990 (U.S. Department of Health and Human Services 1995). Funding for community based programs also increased during this time period and continues to do so into the 1990s. The managed health care movement and the advocacy of managed health care principles has also increased. The specific regulatory agencies and standards that apply to managed health care will be discussed later.

Unfortunately, another repercussion of the downsizing of state hospitals and the reduction of available beds has been an increase in the number of mentally ill individuals in the nation's jails and prisons. The Bureau of Criminal Justice Statistics estimates that among the approximately 1.7 million individuals residing in the nation's jails and prisons, 16 to 25 percent have serious and persistent mental illness (U.S. Department of Justice 1997). This increase in the number of mentally ill individuals in our jails and prisons who require screening, evaluation, and crisis intervention services, as well as long-term mental health management services, has resulted in additional budget allocations for health care generally and mental health care specifically in correctional facilities. Associated with this need for increased funding has been the development of more public-private partnerships in correctional facilities through managed care organizations providing services to detainees and inmates with mental illness.

There is a growing need for appropriate mental health services for children, adolescents, and their families. This specific population is frequently excluded in the planning for mental health services. The provision of care in the least restrictive environment as well as the efforts to avoid the stigmatization of children and adolescents as having serious mental illness are factors that influence the development of services. In most states inpatient services are typically small units whose mission must include consideration of the age of the child or adolescent who is to be admitted to the program. Typically, inpatient units provide services to children under the age of six, from the age of six to twelve, or from the age of thirteen to eighteen. Community/residential services, however, are an entirely different matter. A number of states do not provide significant community or residential services within their jurisdictional boundaries. Frequently, states and mental health systems contract with other mental health care providers based in other states that have residential facilities to provide care and treatment for the seriously emotionally disturbed child or adolescent. A number of the children and adolescents in these programs have some relationship with the juvenile justice system, and may be in such facilities because of neglect or delinquency that may be related to their serious emotional disturbances. The services for the individual child/adolescent may be geographically distant from the services provided for the families who may remain in the original jurisdiction. Therefore, the integration of mental health care services, is quite challenging and requires special considerations.

Other legal mandates such as the Americans with Disabilities Act (1996) and the Prison Litigation Reform Act (1996) are federal mandates that require provision for service to specific populations. The Americans with Disabilities Act requires reasonable accommodation by employers for employees who may have significant mental illness with appropriate allowances for the provision of service. While the Prison Litigation Reform Act strives to reduce the number of frivolous lawsuits by incarcerated inmates, service provision is also influenced by the Americans with Disabilities Act, which has been determined by the federal government to also apply to prisoners with regard to their health and mental health needs.

The development of managed care and managed care principles, particularly those applicable to mental health services, has generated more discussion and debate in the mental health community than any other single issue in the last decade. The provision of the appropriate level of service in a timely manner with cost containment factors as a primary consideration has resulted in a number of approaches to managed care in mental health systems. Funding for these approaches includes capitation of services, carve-outs for mental health services from general health services, development of medical necessity criteria, and great concerns with regard to parity and choice for mental health services as compared with general health services. A number of professional mental health associations and consumer rights organizations have lobbied Congress vigorously for consideration of these factors, particularly with regard to parity, availability of services, and choice regarding providers of service. The result has been President Clinton's establishment of a Patient's Bill of Rights that has particular implications for these stated issues in the pursuit of mental health services by consumers. These factors must also be considered in the planning and implementation of administrative components of mental health services.

Structure of Mental Health Service Delivery Systems

Mental health service delivery systems are configured in a variety of ways. Some are owned, operated, and in part regulated by the state or federal government. Others have state or federal government oversight but are operated by private not-for-profit providers. Others may be private entities that are for profit, but must meet state, federal, and other regulatory requirements. And, still others may be a combination of these models. **The basic structure, however, tends to be as indicated by the following diagram:**

Governing Body
Administration Oversight
Professional Oversight
Providers of Services
Consumers of Services

Each of these levels represents particular responsibilities and authorities and may have a series of advisory boards, consumer or citizen participation, academic affiliations, and, of course, regulatory review. The governing body of the organization is the entity that is responsible for provision of fiscal and human resources, and approval and endorsement of the system's mission and goals. The administrative oversight component is responsible for the operations of the mental health system and is the mechanism for conveying the needs of recipients and providers of care to the resource allocators, i.e., the governing body. The professional staff organization component is responsible for establishing the standards of practice, and reviewing and assuring the competence and proper service provision by the direct service providers. It is also responsible for communicating the needs of the providers such as sufficient staff numbers, proper qualifications, and specificity regarding implementation of the mission to the administrative and governing components of the system. The direct providers of service are responsible for the day-to-day assessment, evaluation, treatment and/or referral of individuals who come into the service provision system as well as continuing care and appropriate discharge from the system when services are no longer required. Fortunately, for the mental health community at all levels of these components—consumers, clients, patients—recipients of care are having a greater voice in the actual operations, management, mission, and vision for the service delivery system. Consumers are also gaining more input and participation in the standards of practice setting mechanisms of professional organizations and of the regulatory standards that are being promoted and implemented by regulatory agencies in their review criteria. This basic structure lends itself to specific levels of regulatory review.

Types of Regulatory Review

1. Compliance with State and Federal Law Is a Fundamental Requirement of All Mental Health Systems. Administrators must be aware of the local, state, and applicable federal laws that are relative to the mental health services delivery system in their locale. Licensure of the facilities by the state as well as requirements for licensure of practitioners and verifications of such licensure is an integral part of the administrative responsibilities.

2. Payers of Service Delivery. Those who are responsible for payment for services to allow the system to continue to function is a second level of regulatory review. Payment may be through the federal government by way of the Health Care Financing Administration (Medicare and Medicaid) or other federal payments. Such payments may be through the state as part of the state budget with appropriate approval by the state legislature.

Health maintenance organizations, preferred provider organizations, and managed care organizations represent a third level of payment. These components are usually paid directly by the state or federal government for services provided via contracts for the level and number of services, based on payment formulas. Private insurers and direct payment from recipients of care are the fourth level of payers for service delivery.

3. Recipients of Service. The roles and participation of consumers, clients, patients, survivors, and other recipients of service engaged in direct payment or in payment via third parties has been greatly accelerated due to the consumer movement within the United States for a voice in the delivery of health care services generally. Consumer organizations, such as the National Alliance for the Mentally Ill, have taken the lead in attempting to nationalize standards and to have an impact on the development of professional practice standards as well as regulatory agency standards of care. The federal government has established protection and advocacy components through block grants to each state and jurisdiction of the United States. These agencies provide an oversight component for each mental health service delivery system to assure that services are in compliance with local and federal law and represent good standards of practice.

4. Regulatory Agencies. There are a number of regulatory agencies that have developed their own specific standards and we will discuss these in detail. The agencies that will be specifically discussed include:

A. The Joint Commission on Accreditation of Healthcare Organizations (JCAHO)
B. The Commission on Accreditation of Rehabilitation Facilities (CARF)
C. The National Committee for Quality Assurance (NCQA)
D. The National Commission on Correctional Health Care (NCCHC)
E. The Health Care Financing Administration (HCFA)

5. Professional Certification and Licensure. Professional certification is a process that is administered by professional organizations to validate the training and competence of practitioners in particular specialty areas. These include such organizations as the American Board of Psychiatry and Neurology, the American Psychological Association, the American Nursing Association, the National Association of Social Workers, and other professional groups. It also includes their jurisdictional boundaries, and includes specific licensure for such things as prescribing controlled substances by physicians. This level of regulatory review is at the individual practitioner level and is intended to provide verification that the appropriate training, experience, qualifications, and ongoing competence has been demonstrated by the individual practitioners in the specialty area for the services they are intended to provide.

Mission and Intent of Review Mechanisms

The various agencies that provide accreditation, certification, licensure, and other forms of approval for a particular service provision have their own specific standards and requirements. However, there are some common themes and expectations that apply to nearly all of these agencies and may be listed as follows:

1. Quality Services: All of the regulatory agencies have as part of their mission the provision of quality, that is, services that are reflective of the needs of the recipient of service and are provided by competent practitioners in the most appropriate settings. How each of the regulatory agencies defines quality demonstrates considerable variability and will be discussed as each regulatory agency is profiled.

2. Professional and Administrative Competence: The matter of those who provide service having appropriate licensure, experience, training, and qualifications as well as those administering services having appropriate facilities, funding, insurance, and other elements to best assure professional and administrative competence, is an integral part of all regulatory agencies.

3. Appropriate Range of Services: Largely based on the mission and goals of the particular mental health service delivery system and qualifications and competence of the specific providers, regulatory agencies have standards that apply to assure that the appropriate range of services from intensive acute to continuing/preparation for discharge/referral services is in place. Not only does the appropriate provision of services need to be demonstrated, but mechanisms for referral to services not within the range of services within a particular system must be identified. Further, criteria for discharge from services must be provided.

4. Consumer/Patient Rights: The rights to the provision of care and treatment with dignity in the least restrictive environment and in collaboration with the recipient of care is of particular concern to regulatory agencies. Even the terminology that may be applied by the providers of service or the mental health service delivery system has changed over the years, largely in response to the consumer movement and is becoming more reflective of that movement in standards by various regulatory agencies. The terms *customer, consumer, client, patient, survivor, recipient,* and *resident* apply to those who are on the receiving end of services and may reflect issues of the rights of individuals not only to services but also to dignity and respect.

5. Public Safety: Regulatory agencies are consistent in having standards that have to do with the issues raised here (i.e., consumer or patient rights while in facilities particularly but also in the community). These particular issues of patient rights have been largely generated because of abuses of particular forms of intervention in mental health and other facilities, particularly involving the interaction of staff with consumers as well as the utilization of involuntary interventions. Such interventions include seclusion, restraint, medication given without the patient's consent, and hospitalization or release from hospitalization without the patient's consent. The issue of public safety is reflected in a number of regulatory agencies having to do with the concerns and, at times, contrasting objectives involved in the rights of the individual consumer versus the requirements for public safety in the community or in facilities. The issues of not causing risk of serious harm by persons with mental illness who may have demonstrated dangerous behavior and assuring the safety of consumers in inpatient or residential facilities from other consumers is a part of the public safety requirement demonstrated in a number of regulatory standards.

6. Funding and Resource Allocation: Regulatory agencies have recognized the need for appropriate resources to assure compliance with the mission of the particular mental health service delivery system and/or provider. Particular standards apply to governing body and other resource allocators in a number of regulatory agencies.

7. Measurable Goals and Objectives: The quality assurance/improvement process: All regulatory agencies have standards that apply to the mental health service delivery system reviewing its practices, services, and outcomes. **These standards vary across regulatory agencies but reflect common concerns that the services being provided are: (1) reflective of the mission, goals, and objectives of the system; (2) consistent with the specific needs of the individual consumer; (3) provided in a consistent and appropriate fashion; (4) include a mechanism for measurement, assessment, review, and revision of the services provided; and (5) result in continuation of quality services that are being appropriately delivered and changes in those areas which are substandard or require improvement. The expectation for outcome measures which demonstrate individual recipients of care receive appropriate and timely services in compliance with the regulatory agency's standards and associated state and federal laws span the range of services from intake to discharge. While the implementation of particular quality improvement mechanisms may vary, the expectations that the quality improvement system is effective, demonstrates measurable outcomes, and results in improvement**

in the overall system as well as in individual cases are reflected in specific standards of all regulatory agencies.

8. Accountability: Regulatory agencies have assigned particular standards that are designed to measure accountability at all levels in the service delivery system. This accountability ranges from the direct service component by competent practitioners to the overall fiscal management of facilities and resources by the governing body. The integration of specific system components is also reflected in standards related to accountability.

9. Basic Principles of Regulatory Agencies: A number of very basic principles are reflected in the standards generated by all regulatory agencies. Understanding of these basic principles is necessary for the administrator to both assess his/her own mental health service delivery system but also to begin the process of application for regulatory review. Without a clear understanding of the basic principles, administrators may find themselves failing to demonstrate or document particular elements, which will result in an unfavorable rating by the regulatory agency because of a seriously flawed preparation process. These basic principles of regulatory agencies are those components that the agencies fully expect any mental health service delivery system to demonstrate. They include:

A. Compliance with state and federal law: Any facility that is unlicensed, is not licensed for the population served, or employs practitioners who have not demonstrated current licensure certification or registration in compliance with their own professional organizations, as well as state and federal law, is very likely to receive an unfavorable rating from a regulatory agency.

B. Appropriateness of services to population served: If there are major gaps in services or an inability to provide services responsive to the consumers' needs at the appropriate time, the mental health service delivery system is incomplete and seriously flawed. The provision of services does not have to be on-site or within the particular mental health system, but must be available in a timely manner. A good example of services that must be available, but are not usually included in the mental health system itself, is general surgery and obstetrical services. Most mental health systems do not have their own surgical and/or delivery suites; however, most have an arrangement with a local hospital or other provider for such services. In correctional settings particularly, there may be an absence of on-site medical professionals to provide for emergency treatments on a timely basis. The requirement for such services to be immediately available within the system or by referral to other providers is a necessity from a regulatory perspective.

Similarly, services for children, adolescents, the dually diagnosed (mental illness and mental retardation, mental illness and substance abuse, or mental illness and physical illness) must be accounted for in the mental health system's policies, procedures, and referral practices. The rising need for services specifically designed to facilitate and maintain the health of elderly consumers is becoming an increasing concern to regulatory agencies and such services must be provided directly or by referral.

C. Acknowledgment of the regulatory process and compliance with standards: Not only are policies and procedures and other documents required to demonstrate compliance with the standards, but notification of consumers, and at times the public and/or other regulatory agencies that the mental health system is undergoing a regulatory review, is a requirement of some regulatory agencies. Over the last decade the results of regulatory reviews have become more public. In the past such reviews were seen as the "property" of the particular mental health system reviewed. However, over the past several years, the results of such reviews have become part of the public domain and may be requested by individuals, attorneys in litigation, and other regulatory agencies to review compliance with the standards of a particular regulatory authority. Further, mental health service delivery systems that have applied for regulatory review have been required by some agencies to verify in writing their compliance with standards during particular time frames and under specific conditions.

D. Linkage of process with service delivery and funding: **The process of review by a regulatory agency is a hands-on process which includes on-site review by representatives of that agency. It is not simply a paper review of policies and procedures, clinical records, and other documents to demonstrate compliance with the letter of the standards.** In fact, the regulatory review process frequently includes interviews of recipients and providers of services. It also includes a review of the funding and resource allocation mechanisms and may include direct interviews with administrators, governing body members, and other individuals responsible for resource allocation.

Specific Regulatory Agencies

There are some general points that are common to all regulatory agencies. These important points are:

1. **All regulatory agencies publish standards and/or guidelines to facilitate understanding of their particular accreditation or certification process.**
2. **All regulatory agencies emphasize basic principles including life safety, clinical competence, and patient/client/consumer rights.**
3. **All regulatory agencies define the populations and types of organizations they survey.**
4. **All private regulatory agencies survey facilities by invitation only (initially), and on an as-needed basis should their findings be less than in compliance or acceptable.**
5. **All regulatory agencies engage consultants, surveyors, and/or site visitors to conduct the process of survey and make recommendations to the central governing body of the regulatory agency.**

Given these basic principles, it is important to be able to distinguish the differences between the particular regulatory agencies. We will discuss several agencies to better understand their processes.

1. The Joint Commission on Accreditation of Healthcare Organizations: The Joint Commission on Accreditation of Healthcare Organizations (JCAHO), established in 1951, is a private organization that has as part of its Board of Commissioners a number of agencies and professional groups. The board establishes appropriate standards of care and compliance for JCAHO accreditation. There are a number of components of the organization that focus on specific types of health care services and providers. The Hospital Accreditation Services produces a manual entitled *The Comprehensive Accreditation Manual for Hospitals* (1996). This manual is updated every two years and is intended to provide the appropriate framework for the survey and review of hospitals. Both general hospitals and psychiatric hospitals are covered under this manual, although other manuals may provide specific standards tailored to cover nonhospital components of a larger system. The Joint Commission also has several other components including Behavioral Health Services, which has the *Behavioral Health Services Manual,* and other components that review and survey nursing homes, homecare facilities, laboratory facilities, free-standing clinics, and the most recent addition to the Joint Commission accreditation standards focus, managed care organizations. Each of these components has a respective manual and scoring guidelines. These manuals are specific for those standards that are required of the facilities surveyed; and, the scoring guidelines provide examples of how to achieve full accreditation based on each individual standard. The Joint Commission is the oldest of the private regulatory bodies and is seen by many organizations as the benchmark to reflect quality and appropriate levels of service care delivery. The Joint Commission breaks its standards into three general foci: (1) patient focused functions, (2) organization focused functions, (3) structures with functions. This comprehensive approach includes a review of such areas as assessment and care of patients, patient rights and organizational ethics, patient education, leadership, management of information, improving organizational performance, management of human resources, governance, management of medical staff and nursing, in addition to psycho-social rehabilitative functions. The accreditation process includes the assessment and scoring by surveyors who then report their findings to the central offices for review and consideration for recommendation to the Board of Commissioners of the Joint Commission. The Board of Commissioners "giveth and/or taketh away" accreditation.

2. The Commission on Accreditation of Rehabilitative Facilities (CARF): The Commission on Accreditation of Rehabilitative Facilities was established in 1966 and includes a number of sponsoring and associate members. The sponsoring and associate members are reflective of the professional and other organizations involved with the delivery of rehabilitative services. The CARF publishes the *Standards Manual for Organizations Serving People with Disabilities* and has a number of standards for which compliance is necessary to be accredited by CARF. The Commission on Accreditation of Rehabilitative Facilities establishes accreditation principles, accreditation criteria, and accreditation conditions that are necessary for attainment of this regulatory agency's endorsement. The Commission on Rehabilitative Facilities publishes on an annual basis the number of programs that have been accredited. The CARF essentially focuses on rehabilitative programs including those that are involved with chronic pain management, spinal cord injury, brain injury, outpatient medical rehabilitation, work hardening programs, vocational evaluations, work adjustment, and a number of other vocational, personal, and social adjustment servicces. The Commission on Accreditation of Rehabilitative Facilities states as its mission "to serve as a preeminent standards setting and accrediting body promoting the delivery of quality services to people with disabilities."

3. The National Committee for Quality Assurance (NCQA): The National Committee for Quality Assurance is a relatively new accrediting body establishing standards in 1991. The standards utilized by the National Committee are published as *The Standards for Accreditation of Managed Care Organizations* (1996), which states as its intention "to develop standards that effectively evaluate the structure and function of medical and quality management systems in managed care organizations. The standards of the National Committee have been evolving over the last several years and have expanded to include credentialing, recredentialing, quality improvement, utilization management, members' rights and responsibilities, preventive care service guidelines, and medical records. The NCQA is reported to have delayed implementation of behavioral health care standards beyond 1999."

4. The National Commission on Correctional Health Care (NCCHC): As the name would imply, the National Commission on Correctional Health Care is an accrediting body that essentially reviews health and mental health services in jails and prisons. This accrediting agency was formed largely with the support of the American Psychiatric Association and other professional organizations who are members of its advisory board. As with other agencies, the advisory board is comprised of professional and other organizations involved in the delivery of health care and/or management of the population in receipt of health care. The National Commission also has published standards regarding health and mental health which are specific in that they attempt to balance the individual needs and rights of detainees and prisoners in correctional systems with those security and custodial concerns relative to the proper operation of a correction facility (National Commission on Correctional Health Care 1996). The standards of the NCCHC are applicable to jail programs whose central focus may be on screening, crisis intervention, and referral for more intensive services through prison services. These services may include a wide variety of in-house as well as contractual services for the provision of health and mental health care to long-term residents.

5. The Health Care Financing Administration (HCFA): Of the regulatory agencies reviewed, the Health Care Financing Administration is the only regulatory agency that is sponsored by the federal government (U.S. Department of Health and Human Services Health Care Financing Administration 1997). This agency is intricately involved in the review, evaluation, and regulation of hospitals and other programs that receive Medicare and/or Medicaid funding. Medicare funding, Title XVIII, applies to individuals who are sixty-five years and older, children, and the severely disabled and identifies distinct parts of health care organizations that may provide care to these populations. Medicaid, Title XIX, is designed for the support of care to the indigent and requires a state-federal match of funding. In the 1970s there was an expansion of Medicaid funding for community services and in the 1990s the establishment of a disproportionate share that has largely to do with provision of care in state psychiatric hospitals. The HCFA certification process involves there being a visit by HCFA surveyors to review the quality and appropriateness of care in the service delivery system. There is a relationship between HCFA and the Joint Commission on Accreditation of Healthcare Organizations that allows that facilities that are accredited by JCAHO may be given deemed status such that HCFA will accept certain findings and recommendations made by JCAHO. Even with deemed status the Health Care Financing Administration focuses largely on issues of staffing and medical records documentation to demonstrate the provision of active treatment for individuals that may fall under the Medicare or Medicaid programs. Over the last several years there have been a number of HCFA waivers to allow for the provision of services to other than traditional populations. These waivers have included 1,915 waivers which allow freedom of choice regarding health care provider and 1,115 waivers which allow redefinition of policy and programming to include nontraditional populations. While there are some distinctions between the particular provisions of Medicare (i.e., a fully federally funded program with part A, payment for hospital care, and part B [an optional component], payment to physicians for some health needs including a 50 percent copay) and Medicaid (which requires a 50/50 federal-to-state match, which may vary with the relative wealth of the particular state), the actual survey process is quite similar. The process as noted includes application of particular HCFA standards to the facility being surveyed and consideration of other regulatory body findings, most specifically, the Joint Commission on Healthcare Organizations.

Essential Components for Review by Regulatory Agencies

As can be observed from the above common and distinct characteristics of regulatory bodies, definition and understanding of the particular mission, vision, and population served by a specific organization are most important in preparing for a regulatory agency review. **There are some very basic principles one should follow in preparation for any regulatory review agency, and they may be referred to as Patterson's Top Ten Considerations for Preparation.**

1. Know your agency and population. It is essential that health care administrators have a complete understanding of the agency in which they serve, the requirements of that agency, and the population served.

2. Know state, local, and federal laws that are applicable to your facility and its practitioners. Quite clearly licensure requirements must precede any review by regulatory agencies rather than subsequently achieved as a condition of accreditation or certification. In fact, licensure of facilities for their recipient populations as well as licensure of practitioners as competent providers is necessary prior to any site visit.

3. Know the manuals and standards of the appropriate regulatory agency. While it is essential that policy and procedure manuals be written to provide direction and instruction for clinicians, administrators, support staff, and volunteers within an organization, the health care administrator must understand and be very familiar with the appropriate standards that are applicable to their organization. A very important rule of thumb is to write policies and procedures that are reflective of the agency organization and then to review the standards and make a match between operational practices and standards for regulatory organizations.

4. Preparation for regulatory agency review is an ongoing, year-round activity. Organizations that are successful in satisfying the requirements of regulatory agencies, do so largely because they practice their standards on an ongoing basis. A major pitfall of many organizations is to begin the process of survey preparation a short time before a survey. Many times, these organizations fail because they do not demonstrate competent knowledge of the standards or a track record to support ongoing functioning.

5. Define your organization for the regulatory agency. It is important to remember that surveyors and central office staff of regulatory agencies prior to survey have very little specific information as to who you are or what you do. In order to establish your identity and make it clear that you are dedicated to your mission and vision, your organization must define itself. This means that policy and procedures, and mission and vision statements are quite clear with regard to the actual operations and planned operations for the organization.

6. Documentation is key. Many organizations that do a reasonable job fail in regulatory agency review because their documentation simply does not satisfy the standards and does not reflect the level of service they provide. It is extremely important that documentation be sufficient to demonstrate the organization's performance.

7. Ongoing training, education, and supervision are essential. The ongoing training, education, and supervision of the workforce (i.e., the human resources component of an organization) is extremely important. As standards change, as quality of services change, and as the standard of care for particular levels of services evolves, the organization must demonstrate that it is current, that is, not practicing an outdated form of service delivery.

8. Understand and present the organization's commitment to total quality management, quality improvement, quality assurance, and improving organization performance. All of these are terms that are particularly relevant to demonstrate how the organization looks at itself . . . that the organization establishes criteria, indicators, and other measures of its successes and failures to better allow the organization to evolve and most importantly to deliver an adequate, if not optimum, level of service. These practices must be ongoing and should not be determined by the timing of a site visit.

9. Be prepared for the survey process. This is an important component of any survey by regulatory agencies, that is, to be prepared for the survey itself. While a great deal of preparation may go into the writing of documents, training of staff, and even improvement of the physical plant with fresh paint and furnishings, many facilities fail to recognize the need for a smooth process for survey. A smooth process means starting on time, being familiar with the requirements of a survey team, providing documents, medical records, and other information necessary to facilitate the process, and informing staff and recipients of care that the process is occurring. This preparation can be achieved in a number of ways but should certainly be in place and ready for activation at the time of the actual survey.

10. There should be no surprises. One of the most important principles for achieving regulatory agency acceptability is the ability to demonstrate to the regulatory agency that you have a process of service delivery, documentation, review of services, improvement of services, and sharing of information that greatly reduces the likelihood of surprises during day-to-day operations or the course of survey. The properly prepared mental health administrator will not be surprised by: (1) opening doors and discovering physical plant deterioration; (2) reviewing personnel records and discovering unlicensed or incompetent practitioners; (3) reviewing unusual events such as deaths, infection outbreaks, or other patient or client care outcomes that have not been thoroughly reviewed during the facility's regular course of review of services and operations; and (4) simple mechanical operations such as locks that do not open, elevators that do not work, and fire alarms, smoke detectors, and other life safety mechanisms that are not functional. There should be an ongoing process that allows for the early and timely detection of such deficiencies and appropriate reparations that are not dependent on a survey process.

These principles are extremely important in the preparation for any regulatory agency review and/or visit. The preparation for such a review or visit may be influenced by a number of activities. These activities include a regular ongoing committee or group process that reviews important aspects of service delivery and pays particular attention to high-risk and high-volume services. In addition, the role of consultants and obtaining information from other systems or facilities that have a similar mission is extremely important in not reinventing the wheel but, rather, gaining from the experience and expertise of others who do similar work. This gaining of expertise and experience from others should then be incorporated into the mission and vision for the specific facility to best maximize the benefit of such systematic review.

Further, the role of consultants may be ongoing for newly developing or evolving programs but also may include target teams, that is, members of the clinical, professional, administrative, and support staff of the facility as well as consultants from outside of the facility to conduct mock surveys.

Mock surveys are short-term surveylike processes to take a snapshot of the facility for a three to five day period that is intended to replicate as much as possible the actual survey process. One of the most important things about any mock survey process is to conduct such a survey as closely as can be to a real survey. That is, members of the survey team should not be engaged in collegial bantering with staff members that may be very well-known to them but, rather, should appear at the appointed time and appointed place as if they are visitors from afar. Such visitors from afar or survey tourists should conduct themselves according to their understanding of the standards and set a schedule that is as closely mirroring what should be expected in a regular survey event. This process should include not only the review of materials and documents but also the on-site touring of facility programs and the face-to-face interviewing techniques utilized by surveyors with staff and with recipients of care. There should be particular attention to the physical plant, the ease of accessibility and availability of services, and the skills and competence of the staff of the facility. This includes not only a review of clinical staff who may know their business but also of their awareness of the actual survey process. This includes the ability to define the facility operations, mission, goals, and vision and to demonstrate an awareness and, in fact, eagerness to achieve regulatory body compliance. Attitudes are as important during the survey process as they are in the delivery of health care services. While competence of practitioners must be assured, competence alone is not enough.

The health care administrator should be clear in understanding the role of regulatory bodies in the proper administration of a mental health care service delivery program. Such understanding reflects awareness of the level of operations, service delivery, and human resources, and knowledge of the survey process standards and requirements as well as specific issues relevant to service delivery for similar patient or client populations. All of these factors come together under the direction of the health care administrator.

Finally, **to be a successful administrator requires not only proper service delivery, but the assurance that the services will continue.** The necessity of achieving regulatory compliance with the appropriate regulatory agencies is in part to demonstrate competent and appropriate service delivery but also to facilitate the ongoing funding of systems and recognition of systems as important components of governmental or private organizational agencies to best serve the population identified. This overview of regulatory agencies and principles applicable to regulatory requirement satisfaction is intended to assist the health care administrator in performing his/her duties to optimal degrees and to provide the system with the leadership necessary to continue the delivery of services to those in need.

GLOSSARY

ADA The Americans with Disabilities Act is an act established in 1996 that provided specific guidelines reflective of the rights of disabled persons and the responsibilities of individuals and systems regarding those rights

The Association of Medical Superintendents of American Institutions for the Insane An organization founded in 1844 that later became the American Psychiatric Association

Asylum A place of refuge and shelter

CARF The Commission on Accreditation of Rehabilitation Facilities is a national not-for-profit organization that establishes standards and accredits organizations serving persons with disabilities

Carve-out A process of segregating a portion of a population for purposes of providing medical and health services through an organization different from the customary services delivery system

Community Mental Health Centers Act A federal act established in 1963 mandating the creation of community mental health systems throughout the country. Funding was provided for the construction of community mental health centers

The Comprehensive Accreditation Manual for Hospitals The accreditation manual utilized by the JCAHO for surveys specific to hospitals

Deemed status A circumstance in which the HCFA considers and accepts certain findings and recommendations made by JCAHO in its survey process

Funding sources Any component of the systems that provides monies or fiscal support for services

Governing body That part of an organization that is responsible for attaining, insuring, and distributing resources, as well as endorsing the system's mission, vision, and goals

HCFA The Health Care Financing Administration is that federal agency that is responsible for monitoring and evaluating programs that receive Medicare of Medicaid funding

HMO A health maintenance organization provides medical and health services under contract to a general population under a capitated payment plan

Insanity A legal term defined by specific criteria to describe a condition in which a mental disease or disorder has been determined to have legally mitigating significance regarding criminal responsibility

JCAHO The Joint Commission on Accreditation of Healthcare Organizations is a private not-for-profit organization that establishes national standards and provides an accreditation process for health care organizations at the request of those organizations

Lunatic An antiquated term meaning a mentally deranged person

Managers of services Individuals who are responsible for the overall operations of a particular mental health system

MCO A managed care organization is an organization that contracts to provide health services to a specific population in a specific manner for a specific reimbursement amount or fee

Measurements of quality The process of demonstrating the delivery of appropriate and competent health care services is a systemized, measurable format. A number of terms have been used through the years to reinforce the principles of measures of quality, including *quality assurance, quality improvement, total quality management,* and *improving organizations' performance,* as well as others

Medicaid The federal program Title XIX designed for funding health and mental health programs for the indigent

Medicare The federal program Title XVIII for funding health and mental health services for individuals who are sixty-five years and older, children, and the severely disabled

Mission The stated purpose and intent of a health care delivery system

NAMI The National Alliance for the Mentally Ill is an organization of consumers, families, and concerned community members to promote the appropriate care and treatment of the mentally ill, not the emotionally disturbed

NCCHC The National Committee for Correctional Health Care is an accrediting body that reviews the health and mental health services in jails and prisons and provides accreditation to programs meeting its standards

NCQA The National Committee for Quality Assurance is an organization that established standards for the accreditation of managed care organizations

Needs assessment An analysis of the specific requirements for health care of a given population

PLRA The Prison Litigation Reform Act is a federal mandate of 1996 defining the rights of prisoners to instigate litigation against correctional providers with guidelines for the appropriate mechanisms for resolution of complaints or concerns

PPO A preferred provider organization is an organization that contracts to provide medical and health services to a specific population using specific providers with whom it generally contracts for services

"Principles of Practice" A treatise written by Thomas Kirkbride in 1876 describing twenty criteria he considered necessary for the proper operation and utilization of mental institutions and hospitals

Professional certification A mechanism whereby professional organizations certify that members of the organization are competent practitioners in particular specialty areas

Providers of services Individuals who are responsible for the actual delivery or interface with recipients of services, such as medical, mental health, or other practitioners

Recipients of services Any individuals who are receiving services from providers and who may be referred to by a number of terms, including *consumers, customers, clients, patients, recipients, survivors, the insane, inmates,* and other terms particular to specific systems and criteria

Regulatory standards Those specific elements that define the acceptable criteria to meet the requirements of a regulatory agency

Restraints Any mechanical device usually made of leather, plastic, or metal used to restrain an individual's movement. The use of restraints may be by means of restraint of free movement of the limbs, restraint of movement in a chair, or restraint of movement to a bed

Seclusion Use of a locked room from which an individual is unable to exit without the assistance of another individual with a key or other control of the locked door

Stakeholders Individuals or groups that are involved with the system at any level, including recipients, providers, managers, resource allocators, and others who have a vested interest in the service delivery system

Statutory or legal requirements Services or other requirements such as licensure, insurance, and appropriate funding that are mandated by state or federal law

The Standards for Accreditation of Managed Care Organizations The accreditation manual utilized by NCQA for accreditation of managed care organizations

The Standards for Health Services in Jails The manual published by the NCCHC for accreditation of health and mental health services in jails

Standards Manual for Organizations Serving People with Disabilities The accreditation manual utilized by CARF in surveying facilities that applied for accreditation by CARF

REFERENCES

Americans with Disabilities Act (ADA). 1990. U.S.C. 12101 et seq.

Commission on Accreditation of Rehabilitation Facilities Standards. 1998. *Standards Manual for Organizations Serving People with Disabilities.* Tucson, AZ: Commission on Accreditation of Rehabilitation Facilities Standards.

Freedman, A., H. Kaplan, and B. Sadock. 1976. *Comprehensive Textbook of Psychiatry.* 2nd ed. Baltimore, MD: Williams and Wilkins.

Grob, Gerald N. 1994. *The Mad among Us: A History of the Care of America's Mentally Ill.* Boston: Harvard University Press.

Joint Commission on Accreditation of Healthcare Organizations (JCAHO). 1996. *The Comprehensive Accreditation Manual for Hospitals.* Oakbrook Terrace, IL: JCAHO.

McKown, Robin M. 1961. *Pioneers in Mental Health.* New York: Dodd, Mead.

National Commission on Correctional Health Care. 1996. *Standards for Health Services in Jails.* Chicago: National Commission on Correctional Health Care.

National Committee for Quality Assurance. 1998. *Standards for the Accreditation of Managed Care Organizations.* Annapolis Junction, MD: National Committee for Quality Assurance Publications Center.

Prison Litigation Reform Act (PLRA). 1996. 18 U.S.C. 3626 et seq.

U.S. Department of Health and Human Services. 1995. *Mental Health, United States 1994.* Rockville, MD: Substance Abuse and Mental Health Services Administration, U.S. Department of Health and Human Services.

U.S. Department of Health and Human Services. 1997. *State Operations Manual, Appendix AA: Psychiatric Hospitals Interpretive Guidelines and Survey Procedures. Pub 7, Rev. 280.* Washington, DC: Health Care Financing Administration.

U.S. Department of Justice. 1997. *Bureau of Justice Statistics Bulletin: Prison and Jail Inmates at Mid-Year, 1996. NCJ-162843.* Washington, DC: U.S. Department of Justice.

CHAPTER 5

Mental Health Law

Charles L. Scott, M.D.

> Wherever a doctor cannot do good he must be kept from doing harm.
> —Hippocrates c. 460–377 B.C.E.

The interface between mental health and the law has grown significantly during the last fifty years. With the advent of managed care, patient's rights and increasing malpractice claims, the provider cannot operate in a vacuum. The knowing autonomous. clinician free from regulatory restraint no longer exists. **As a result, mental health administrators must be familiar with the laws that govern their clinicians' care.**

Learning objectives presented in this chapter are:

- Basic legal concepts
- Common areas of mental health law
- Practical guidelines in the management of key legal issues that arise in the provision of mental health care

The information in this chapter is organized into a series of topics relevant to the administration and delivery of mental health care, as follows:

- Overview of Legal Concepts
- Medical Malpractice
- Malpractice and Suicide
- Managing the Dangerous Patient
- Civil Commitment
- Informed Consent
- Right to Treatment
- Right to Refuse Treatment
- Right to Die
- Confidentiality

Managed Care
Minor's Rights and Health Care

Special features include:

Citation of legal cases related to the provision of mental health care
Practical summary guidelines on managing complex medical legal issues
Case examples and analyses

General Legal Concepts

A knowledge of general legal concepts assists the administrator in both the provision of mental health treatment and in the understanding of medical legal disputes that may arise. In the United States the governmental body authorized to resolve disputes according to law is a court. Criminal courts oversee disputes between a person and the state whereas civil courts oversee disputes between two citizens. In both of these settings, the trial court decides controversies based on facts and procedures and appellate courts review the decisions of the trial courts. Some disputes may be filed in criminal and/or civil courts.

Tort law governs the legal resolution of complaints regarding medical treatment. A **tort** is a civil wrong. Tort law seeks to financially compensate individuals who have been injured or who have suffered losses due to the conduct of others. Torts are typically divided into one of three categories: (1) **intentional torts;** (2) **negligence;** and (3) **strict liability.** Intentional torts involve actions where an individual either intends harm or knows that harm may result from their behavior (Schubert 1996:491). Examples of intentional torts in mental health include assault (an attempt to inflict bodily injury), battery (touching without consent), false imprisonment, and violation of a person's civil rights. A malpractice suit for the sexual exploitation of a patient is commonly forwarded under the intentional tort of assault and battery. Intentional torts may not be covered under malpractice insurance.

Negligent torts result when a person's behavior unintentionally causes an unreasonable risk of harm to another. Medical malpractice is based on the theory of negligence. **Four elements required to establish malpractice include the following:** (1) there must be an established duty between the practitioner and patient; (2) the practitioner demonstrates a dereliction of this duty by an action or lack of action; (3) the patient suffers physical or emotional damages; (4) the practitioner's dereliction of duty is the proximate cause of the patient's injury (Simon 1987:443).

Strict liability imposes liability on defendants without requiring "any proof of lack of due care." The most common example of strict liability is harm caused to an individual resulting from a product proven to be unreasonably dangerous and defective (Schubert 1996:537–41). Plaintiffs have unsuccessfully attempted to apply strict liability doctrine against physicians. In the case of *Hoven v Kelble* (Wisconsin 1977) a plaintiff alleged that strict liability should apply against the defendant doctor whose "defective product" was his provision of medical care. The court refused to impose strict liability on the physician or hospital due to the "unknown costs and inability to assess the results" from such a decision. The court, however, recognized the possibility of applying strict liability to the provision of medical care in the future (Boumil and Elias 1995:230–32).

The standard of proof required in weighing evidence in court varies according to the issue involved. The highest standard is "beyond a reasonable doubt," which represents a certainty of approximately 90 percent or greater. The certainty for the standard of "clear and convincing" is between 70 percent and 80 percent whereas "preponderance of the evidence" is greater than 50 percent. In criminal cases the highest beyond a reasonable doubt standard is required as personal liberty with possible incarceration is at stake. Civil cases involve the potential loss of money not freedom and therefore use the less stringent standard of preponderance of the evidence. Therefore, malpractice can be established if it is more likely than not that the defendant was negligent. The clear and convincing evidence standard is used in civil cases where personal losses greater than money may be involved. Examples include civil commitment and the termination of parental rights.

Medical Malpractice

The four elements required to establish medical malpractice are commonly known as the "four *D*s." To review, these include a **Dereliction** of **Duty** that **Directly** results in **Damages.** A **duty** is most commonly established when the patient seeks treatment and treatment is provided. The provision of services do not require the patient's presence and can extend to assessment and treatment provided over the telephone. Situations where a duty may exist even without the consent of the patient include: (1) emergency treatment of an unconscious individual; (2) treatment of an individual found incompetent to consent to care; (3) third parties at risk for a communicable disease; and (4) third parties at risk of harm from dangerous patients.

Dereliction of duty is usually the most difficult component of negligence to establish. Dereliction of duty is divided into acts of commission (providing substandard care) and acts of omission (failure to provide care). Acceptable care does not have to be perfect care but that provided by a reasonable practitioner. This standard requires that the provider exercise, in both diagnosis and treatment, "that reasonable degree of care which a reasonably prudent person or professional should exercise in same or similar circumstances" (Black 1979). Two aspects of causation generally cited as establishing negligence include the foreseeability of the bad outcome or the clinician's role in directly causing the harm.

Expert witnesses are usually required to establish both the standard of care and any alleged deviation. No expert witness is required when the care provided is so outrageous that even a lay person could recognize substandard treatment. This situation is referred to as ***res ipsa loquitur*** and is literally translated as " the thing speaks for itself." Amputating the wrong leg while a patient is under anesthesia represents a classic *res ipsa loquitur* case. Components of a *res ipsa loquitur* case include: (1) harm rarely occurs in the absence of negligence; (2) the situation causing the bad outcome is under the exclusive control of the provider; (3) the patient did not contribute to the bad outcome; and (4) only the defendants have access to information concerning what occurred (Resnick 1997).

Damages that result from negligence are divided into three categories. Actual damages are the costs for the expenses directly involved in treating the injury and lost wages. Compensatory damages seek to financially compensate the individual for pain and suffering. Punitive damages seek to punish the wrongdoer and are usually awarded when the provider intended to harm the patient.

Malpractice and Suicide

The possibility of a patient committing suicide represents one of the greatest emotional and legal concerns for clinicians and administrators. This concern is realistic in view of the fact that 10 to 15 percent of patients with major psychiatric disorders will die by suicide (Brent, Kupfer, Bromet, and Dew 1988:353–85). Lawsuits involving suicide generally include one of three scenarios: (1) an inpatient suicide where the facility and its providers provide inadequate care or supervision; (2) a recently discharged patient who commits suicide; or (3) an outpatient who commits suicide (VandeCreek and Knapp 1987).

Suicidality is the most common reason for inpatient psychiatric hospitalization. (Friedman 1989:379–402). When a patient is admitted due to feelings of self-harm, the clinician is on notice that the patient is at an increased risk for suicidal behavior. Nearly one-third of inpatient suicides result in a lawsuit against the hospital (Litman 1982). Eight common allegations for malpractice following an inpatient suicide include: (1) failure to diagnose or foresee the suicide; (2) failure to control, supervise, or restrain; (3) failure to adequately evaluate suicidal intent; (4) failure to provide appropriate pharmacotherapy; (5) failure to provide adequate monitoring; (6) failure to gather an adequate history; (7) failure to remove potentially harmful items such as belts or shoelaces, or lack of supervision of such items; and (8) failure to provide the patient a safe, secure environment. Malpractice actions often include the hospital in addition to the care providers. For example, when the hospital is aware of the patient's suicidal tendencies, then the hospital assumes the duty to prevent the patient from inflicting harm (Robertson 1988).

Common scenarios resulting in malpractice suits for outpatient suicides include: (1) failure to evaluate the need for pharmacotherapy or inappropriate pharmacotherapy; (2) failure to hospitalize; (3) failure to maintain appropriate clinician-patient relationships, (4) failure in supervision or consultation; (5) failure to assess suicide risk at intake or during treatment; (6) failure to secure previous records; (7) failure to diagnose; (8) failure to safeguard the outpatient environment; and (9) failure to document clinical judgment (Bongar, Maris, Berman, and Litman 1998:14–24).

Clinicians and hospital administrators can take precautionary measures to decrease both the risk of a successful suicide and a malpractice action. To minimize liability:

1. **Conduct a thorough assessment of suicide risk factors and document this analysis in the patient's chart.**
2. **Adhere to written hospital policies regarding the management of suicidal patients.**
3. **Attempt to secure and review past treatment records.**
4. **Consider obtaining a second opinion consultation in difficult cases.**
5. **Document ongoing suicide assessments and treatment plans.**

The Dangerous Patient

The dangerous patient represents a risk of harm to others or to property. *Tarasoff v Regents of California* (1976) is the landmark case that extended the duty of outpatient therapists to protect third parties of potential harm. The California Court of Appeals held that,

> when a therapist determines, or pursuant to the standards of his profession should determine that his patient presents a serious danger of violence to another, he incurs an obligation to use reasonable care to protect the intended victim against such danger. The discharge of this

> duty may require the therapist to take one or more of various steps. Thus, it may call for him to warn the intended victim, to notify police, or to take whatever steps are reasonably necessary under the circumstances.

Although the Tarasoff case extended the duty of the clinician to protect an identifiable victim from a patient, some state courts have extended this duty even when there is no identifiable victim (*Lipari v Sears* 1980). A further extension includes psychiatric patients who harm others in automobile accidents (*Naidu v Laird* 1988). In Vermont mental health professionals are potentially liable when their patient's behavior results in destruction of property (*Peck v Counseling Service of Addington County* 1985).

Despite the difficulty in predicting future violence, mental health practitioners are often asked to assess the potential dangerousness of their patients. Rather than attempting to forecast a specific event, psychiatrists should conduct a violence risk assessment (Wack 1993). In assessing the risk of violence, the clinician should carefully review any past history of violence. In general, the best predictor of future violence is a past history of violence (Klassen 1988). Collateral information useful in reviewing previous violent acts include police reports, information from family members, previous hospital records, as well as military and school records. Other risk factors for violence include the presence of psychosis (particularly paranoia), drug and/or alcohol abuse and access to weapons.

Hospital administrators can advise clinicians of various alternatives when managing potentially dangerous patients. These options include notification of the third party and the police, hospitalization of the patient, removal of weapons, increasing the frequency of outpatient visits, involving supportive family members, altering the type of treatment provided, and adjusting medications. **Strategies to reduce malpractice risk in working with potentially violent patients include:**

> 1. **Keeping current regarding the literature on violence risk factors and assessment.**
> 2. **Attempting to obtain all relevant data to include past records.**
> 3. **Documenting reasoning to include a risk benefit analysis regarding patient management.**
> 4. **Knowing the specific state Tarasoff doctrine and case law regarding any requirement of notification of third parties or police.**
> 5. **Closely monitoring and documenting supervision of those who treat potentially violent patients under your guidance.**
> 6. **Obtaining a second opinion in complex or difficult cases. (Resnick and Scott 1997:478)**

Civil Commitment

Two underlying legal doctrines have historically guided involuntary hospitalization. The first doctrine is known as ***parens patriae,*** which is literally translated as the "father of the country." Under this approach, the state makes the decision to hospitalize the patient based upon what the state believes is in the patient's best interest. The second approach is known as **police power.** Here the government hospitalizes the patient to protect society or to protect the patient from self-harm. Most commitment statutes require that a person be mentally ill and dangerous thus combining elements of both doctrines (Appelbaum and Gutheil 1991).

Three general populations subject to civil commitment include persons with mental illness, the developmentally disabled/mentally retarded, and addicts. Nearly two-thirds of states have commitment statutes authorizing the institutionalization of persons addicted to alcohol or drugs. The majority of states also have separate statutes regarding the commitment procedures of individuals found not guilty by reason of insanity and the transfer of prisoners to mental hospitals (Hermann 1997:142–83).

Since the 1960s the pendulum has shifted away from the *parens patriae* model toward patient autonomy. As a consequence, the majority of state civil commitment statutes require that in addition to being mentally ill, developmentally disabled or addicted, the person must represent a risk of harm to others or to self. Approximately 25 percent of jurisdictions authorize commitment if the person is gravely disabled as evidenced by their inability to meet their basic needs. A significant number of states require either a recent specific overt act or evidence that potential danger to others is imminent. Finally, forty-seven states prohibit institutionalization if a less restrictive alternative is available for the patient (Hermann 1997:150).

The United States Supreme Court has recognized that civil commitment results in a "massive deprivation of liberty" for the patient (*Humphrey v Cady* 1972). The standard of proof required for involuntary hospitalization was decided by the *U.S. Supreme Court in Addington v Texas* (1979). The U.S. Supreme Court held that due process requires clear and convincing evidence when a person's liberties are deprived as a result of civil commitment. As personal freedom is at stake, this standard of proof is higher than the preponderance of the evidence standard set forth in other civil cases but less stringent than beyond a reasonable doubt used in criminal cases.

The right of those involuntarily committed to receive treatment was raised before the U.S. Supreme Court in the case of *O'Connor v Donaldson* (1975). Mr. Kenneth Donaldson was confined for nearly fifteen years at

Chattahoochee State Hospital without evidence that he was dangerous while hospitalized. He alleged that his constitutional rights were violated due to malpractice and wrongful confinement. The Supreme Court held that "the state cannot constitutionally confine, without more, a nondangerous individual who is capable of surviving safely in freedom by himself or with the help of willing and responsible family members or friends." This statement has been interpreted to imply that a person cannot be involuntary hospitalized against his will without evidence of dangerousness. The Supreme Court chose to address this case as an involuntary treatment case and did not address the issue of whether involuntary hospitalization mandated actual treatment.

Every state allows for emergency detention for an individual who represents a clear danger to self or others. Often family members, friends, or the police initiate the proceedings. Patients are held for a limited period after which they are either released, admitted voluntarily, or civilly committed (Weiner and Wettstein 1993:46). Most states allow the hospital to detain voluntary patients requesting to leave to determine the need for continued hospitalization and civil commitment.

The involuntary hospitalization of minors was addressed by the U.S. Supreme Court in the case of *Parham v J.R.* (1979). In this case Georgia's statutory scheme for the voluntary commitment of juveniles was challenged. The procedure at issue involved parents or guardians hospitalizing children without the involvement of a judge, attorney, or an adversarial hearing. Although the presence of a mental illness suitable for treatment in a hospital was required, no finding of dangerousness was necessary. The U.S. Supreme Court upheld Georgia's scheme for admitting children where the decision to hospitalize was made by the physician and not the court.

States have various forms of outpatient commitment statutes. One type involves the use of outpatient commitment as a less restrictive alternative to inpatient hospitalization. A second form includes preventative outpatient commitment of a patient who may soon meet inpatient commitment criteria if more immediate intervention does not take place. The final type of outpatient commitment is called conditional release. In this setting the individual is placed under certain conditions that, if violated, may result in a return to the hospital (Melton 1997:311–12). Every state requires a commitment hearing and periodic review of the legal status of individuals committed. Most states also provide notice of the hearing, presence of counsel as well as the right of the patient to communicate with persons outside the hospital (Hermann 1997:150–51). Additional safeguards afforded by some states include the right to call and cross examine witnesses, the right to request a jury trial, and the right to have a judge rather than a clinician make the ultimate decision (Melton 1997:314). A few state statutes provide an independent psychiatric examination before the commitment hearing (Weiner and Wettstein 1993:57).

A patient who has been unlawfully committed can bring a civil suit for the intentional tort of false imprisonment. **Guidelines to minimize liability related to involuntary hospitalization include:**

1. **Knowing your state's statute regarding civil commitment criteria.**
2. **Personally examining and attempting to take a history from the patient or significant others.**
3. **Documenting the reasoning governing the need for an involuntary hospitalization versus voluntary hospitalization or outpatient commitment.**
4. **Considering initiating civil commitment proceedings against those patients incompetent to consent for voluntary treatment who require hospitalization.**
5. **Conducting and documenting ongoing reviews regarding the need for continued commitment.**

Informed Consent

In 1914 Justice Benjamin Cardozo articulated an individual's right to govern their own treatment when he wrote, "Every human being of adult years and sound mind has a right to determine what shall be done with his own body" (qtd. in Schloendorff 1914). The evolution of **informed consent** has involved a balance between medical paternalism (what the doctor thinks the patient should know) and autonomy of the patient (what the patient would like to know). Informed consent requires that the individual: (1) be competent; (2) have the necessary information; and (3) make a voluntary decision.

Competency to give informed consent is determined by the patient's decision making capacity involving health care. A finding of incompetency in other areas (such as incompetency to stand trial or to manage financial affairs) does not equate with incompetency to give informed consent for medical care. Adult patients are presumed competent to give informed consent until a judicial determination is made that the person is incompetent.

There is no one standard for determining competency to make health care decisions. One proposed set of criteria requires that the patient have the ability to make choices as well as to understand, reason, and appreciate presented information (Appelbaum and Roth 1982). Drane (1985) has suggested that the determination of competency be considered on a sliding scale. In other words, the standard for determining competency increases with the potential consequences of the patient's decision.

The assessment of incompetency is predicated on deficits in a person's decision-making capacity that result from mental illness or cognitive impairment. The presence of a mental illness or intellectual deficit does not categorically render one incompetent. For example, an individual with a well-circumscribed delusion unrelated to treatment may be competent to decide treatment despite evidence of psychosis.

The second component of informed consent involves disclosure of information to the patient. The practitioner must provide information to the patient regarding the nature of their illness, the risks and benefits of treatment, the risks and benefits of alternate treatments, and the risks of refusing treatment (Meisel, Roth, and Lidz 1977). Two approaches to the provision of this information have developed. The first, outlined in the case of *Natanson v Kline* (1960), is known as the "reasonable medical practitioner standard." Under this standard the information to be provided to the patient is what a reasonable medical practitioner would disclose in similar circumstances. In contrast, the Washington, DC, Court of Appeals articulated the "reasonable person" standard in the case of *Cantebury v Spence* (1972). This standard shifted the control of the information from what the physician thought should be provided to what a patient would want to know. Here the physician must disclose to the patient what a reasonable patient would want to know under a similar situation. The reasonable person standard is the informed consent standard used in the majority of states. Voluntariness is the final component to establish competency to give informed consent. The clinician should examine issues of coercion or undue influence that may affect the patient's decision. Although a clinician may believe a patient is incompetent, a finding of incompetency to consent to medical care is a judicial rather than a medical decision.

There are four situations in which informed consent is not required. These include: (1) a finding of incompetency; (2) a medical emergency; (3) patient waiver (where the patient states he does not want to make the decision); and (4) therapeutic privilege (Meisel 1979). **Therapeutic privilege** allows the clinician to withhold information from the patient when the clinician believes the disclosure would result in obvious harm. The use of therapeutic privilege should be used with caution and not simply to prevent the patient from refusing care.

Courts may treat the failure by the clinician to obtain informed consent as either an assault and battery (intentional torts) or as an act of negligence (unintentional tort). Because battery is an intentional tort, no expert witness testimony is necessary to establish intent. Punitive damages may be awarded if battery is established. In addition, many malpractice insurance claims do not cover intentional torts. If the clinician is sued under a malpractice claim, then an actual injury resulting from a lack of informed consent is required to establish negligence (Hermann 1997). **To manage informed consent issues:**

1. **Assess the patient's competency to consent to care.**
2. **Know your state's standard for the provision of informed consent.**
3. **Document that informed consent was provided to patient to include the reasons for treatment, risks and benefits to treatment, alternatives to treatment, and possible consequences of not receiving treatment.**
4. **Document discussion of tardive dyskinesia with the patient when neuroleptics are prescribed.**
5. **Understand that incompetency is ultimately a judicial rather than a medical decision.**

Right to Treatment

The issue regarding a constitutional right to treatment in a hospital setting generally arises in involuntarily hospitalized patients. Morton Birnbaum, M.D., J.D., proposed the argument that institutionalized persons had a right to treatment and failure to do so would violate the Fourteenth Amendment substantive due process clause of the United States Constitution. Although the United States Supreme Court has never recognized a constitutional right to treatment, this issue has been addressed by lower courts. In *Rouse v Cameron* the Washington, DC, Circuit Court of Appeals recognized a right to treatment for an involuntarily hospitalized patient based on a DC statute. The court held that "the hospital is not obligated to cure or even improve the patient but bona fide efforts to do so must be made; regular review of progress is expected" (*Rouse v Cameron* 1966). The right to treatment for civilly committed patients was acknowledged in *Wyatt v Stickney,* a 1972 case heard by a federal district court. In this case a class-action lawsuit was filed challenging the conditions and lack of treatment provided to involuntarily committed patients. The court held that when patients are involuntarily hospitalized they have a "constitutional right to receive such individual treatment as will give each of them a realistic opportunity to be cured or to improve his or her mental condition." In a later ruling the court held that minimum constitutional standards for adequate treatment included: (1) a humane psychological and physical environment; (2) qualified staff in numbers sufficient to administer adequate treatment; and (3) individualized treatment plans. In *Wyatt v*

Aderholt the mentally retarded were found to have a right to habilitation that will give them a realistic opportunity to lead a meaningful life and return to society. In 1974 the Fifth Circuit Court of Appeals held that the Fourteenth Amendment guaranteed civil committees a constitutional right to treatment (*Donaldson v O'Connor* 1974). When reviewing this case, the U.S. Supreme Court retreated from the lower court's holding. Instead, the Supreme Court focused on the appropriateness of civilly committing nondangerous individuals. Although the U.S. Supreme Court has not held that involuntary patients have a constitutional right to treatment, it has ruled that involuntarily civilly committed individuals have a right to safe conditions of confinement, freedom from bodily restraint, and adequate habilitation (*Youngberg v Romeo* 1982). The majority of states recognize by statute the right to treatment for both voluntarily and involuntarily hospitalized patients. Difficulties remain in defining what is adequate treatment and how such treatment will be funded (Weiner and Wettstein 1993).

Right to Refuse Treatment

The right of patients who voluntarily sign into a hospital to refuse treatment is well recognized. The controversy regarding the right to refuse treatment centers on those patients who are involuntarily committed. In the vast majority of states, individuals who are involuntarily committed are presumed competent to make treatment decisions including the refusal of treatment (except in emergencies). Three models guide the management of treatment refusals. The first model was established by the case of *Rennie v Klein.* In this case the Third Circuit Court of Appeals recognized that a patient had a right to refuse antipsychotic medication (absent an emergency) based on a constitutionally protected liberty interest. The court also held, however, that dangerous mentally ill patients may be forcibly administered antipsychotics "whenever, in the exercise of professional judgment, such an action is deemed necessary to prevent the patient from endangering himself or others." The court showed deference to the administrative procedures established within the hospital to override the patient's medication refusal. Therefore, clinicians (rather than courts) were allowed to decide whether to override the patient's refusal as long as the decision did not represent a substantial departure from accepted professional judgment, practice, or standards. This model is sometimes referred to as the treatment-driven model.

The second model was outlined in the case of *Rogers v Commissioner.* Here the Massachusetts court held that a competent patient may refuse medication in a nonemergency situation. If the individual is found incompetent by a judge, then the decision to override the patient's treatment refusal is made by the court, not by the treatment team or guardian. The court uses a substituted judgment decision-making process. In an adversarial hearing the judge decides what the incompetent patient would have wanted if competent. Six factors outlined by the judge to be considered included: (1) the patient's previously expressed preference; (2) the patient's religious convictions; (3) the impact on the family from the patient's viewpoint; (4) probable side effects; (5) prognosis with treatment; and (6) prognosis without treatment.

The third model, established in Utah, renders all patients involuntarily hospitalized as incompetent regarding mental health treatment decisions. Therefore, treatment refusals do not require either an internal administrative review or a judicial hearing (Weiner and Wettstein 1993).

Consider the following guidelines when faced with a patient who refuses treatment:

1. **Provide treatment in emergency situations where immediate action is necessary.**
2. **Inquire into the reasons for the patient's treatment refusal and document the patient's response.**
3. **Evaluate risks to patient of treatment refusal.**
4. **Document reasoning for requesting treatment refusal override.**
5. **Learn your state's model for overriding treatment refusal.**
6. **Consider obtaining a second opinion regarding the need for treatment.**
7. **Learn your state's legal guidelines regarding the application of seclusion, restraints, and electroconvulsive therapy.**

Right to Die

The extreme example of treatment refusal is the right of the patient to forego potentially life-sustaining treatment. The refusal of medical care due to religious beliefs was the central issues in the case of *Application of President and Directors of Georgetown College* (1964). In this case Ms. Jones, a twenty-five-year-old mother, lost approximately two-thirds of her blood from an acute GI bleed. As she was a Jehovah's Witness, she and her husband refused to consent for blood transfusions prior to her ulcer surgery. The appellate judge personally interviewed Ms. Jones. When he asked if she would refuse to have the blood transfusions Ms. Jones responded, "Against my will." The judge found Ms. Jones incompetent and ordered the blood transfusion. Part of the judge's decision involved the fact that Ms. Jones had a seven-month-old child who would be without a mother should she die.

The first amendment provides a constitutional right to freedom of religion. The majority of courts will permit treatment refusal based on religious beliefs if the religion is recognized as a legitimate sect and if the refusal is not part of a delusional belief. If the patient is determined incompetent, then a court will often examine any prior treatment refusals and the degree to which the patient strongly practiced their faith when competent (Hermann 1997:195).

The United States Supreme Court addressed competency to end life-sustaining treatment in the case of *Cruzan v Director, Missouri Department of Health* (1990). Nancy Cruzan was a young woman who suffered a car accident that left her in a persistent vegetative state with no meaningful cognitive function (and thereby incompetent). The hospital refused to honor her parent's request to terminate artificial nutrition and hydration. The state of Missouri required clear and convincing evidence of what Nancy would have wanted regarding the withdrawal of her medical treatment when she was competent. The U.S. Supreme Court held that the state of Missouri did not violate the U.S. Constitution by requiring clear and convincing evidence of what the incompetent patient would have wanted when competent. The court also stated, however, that a competent patient can refuse lifesaving nutrition and hydration.

The controversy surrounding the right to die has extended to the right of physicians to assist in the death of their patients. In 1997 two United States Supreme Court decisions (both announced on the same day) addressed the constitutionality of banning physician assisted suicide. In the case of *Washington v Glucksberg* four Washington state physicians stated that they would assist their terminally ill patients in ending their life if Washington state did not have a ban on assisted suicide. These physicians (along with some of their patients) challenged the constitutionality of Washington's ban on grounds that it violated a protected liberty under the Fourteenth Amendment. The Supreme Court held that the ban was not unconstitutional as legitimate government interests were present. Such interests included the prohibition against killing, the deterring of suicide, preserving the medical practitioner's role as healer, and avoiding a move toward euthanasia.

In *Vacco v Quill* (1997) three New York physicians argued that the ban on physician assisted suicide prevented them from prescribing lethal doses of medication for competent terminally ill patients experiencing great physical pain. They asserted that in New York a competent person was allowed to refuse life-sustaining medical treatment that was essentially the same thing as physician assisted suicide. A suit was brought against the New York attorney general alleging that this ban violated the equal protection clause of the Fourteenth Amendment. The U.S. Supreme Court held that the ban on assisted suicide does not violate the equal protection clause. The Court made a clear distinction between allowing a patient to die by removing life support and prescribing medications with the intent to cause the patient's death. In the former, the patient dies as a result of their disease whereas in the latter the patient dies from the administered drugs. Many of the same reasons cited in *Washington v Gluck* for banning physician assisted suicide were also cited in this case. These Supreme Court rulings do not prevent a state from permitting physician assisted suicide. In fact, Oregon allows physician assisted suicide, which has been utilized by patients.

When considering a patient's request to refuse life-sustaining treatment:

1. **Determine the patient's present competency status regarding health care decision-making capacity.**
2. **Know your state statute and/or case law regarding the evidentiary standards for the incompetent patient's right to refuse life-sustaining treatment.**
3. **Know your state's laws regarding the permissibility of physician assisted suicide.**
4. **Determine and review any advance directives and living wills written by the patient.**

Confidentiality

Confidentiality in the medical setting has long been recognized as a fundamental component of the doctor-patient relationship. The Hippocratic oath states, "Whatever in connection with my professional practice, or not in connection with it, I see or hear, in the life of men, which ought not to be spoken of abroad, I will not divulge, as reckoning that all such should be kept secret." Confidentiality differs from privilege. Confidentiality represents the clinician's obligation to keep communication by a patient private. **Privilege** represents the patient's right to bar the clinician from testifying about professional-obtained material in a judicial or parajudicial setting. The term *privilege* has also been called **testimonial privilege** (Appelbaum and Gutheil 1991:4).

Confidentiality may be breached when consent to release information has been obtained. Such consents can be obtained from a legally competent adult, the legal guardian of an incompetent adult, an emancipated minor, the parent of an unemancipated minor, and the executor or administrator of the estate of a deceased person. The clinician can legally breach confidentiality without consent in the following situations: (1) emergencies; (2) civil commitment; (3) notification and protection of third parties from harm; (4) mandated child and elder abuse reporting; and (5) discussion of the case with treating consultants and supervisors. Some state statutes require mandated reporting in cases involving knife and gunshot wounds, the transmission of communicable diseases and the presence of a physical or emotional disorder that could impair the person's driving (Wettstein 1993:201–30). Additional areas in which confidentiality is not expected include forensic and court-ordered evaluations, treatment provided to military personnel, and juvenile court.

The most common exception to the patient's right to waive confidential information involves the patient litigant exception. In the patient litigant exception the patient waives their privilege to confidentiality if their mental health is raised in a lawsuit. Examples include child custody disputes, personal injury actions, malpractice suits against the therapist, disability and workers' compensation claims, and will contests. Whenever a therapist receives a subpoena or is asked to testify regarding a patient of the therapist, the therapist should first notify the patient and the patient's attorney to verify if the privilege has been waived.

In *Jaffe v Redmond* (1996) the United States Supreme Court addressed whether a psychotherapist privilege existed under Rule 501 of the Federal Rules of Evidence. Mary Lu Redmond, a police officer, shot and killed a suspect. Ms. Redmond was subsequently charged with violating the victim's constitutional rights by using excessive force. The officer later participated in counseling sessions with a social worker. Both the social worker and Ms. Redmond refused to turn over the treatment notes to the court. The U.S. Supreme Court held that the conversations between Redmond and her therapist were protected from compelled disclosure. This privilege extends to psychiatrists, psychologists, and licensed social workers who provide psychotherapy. This ruling applies only to federal civil and federal criminal courts.

Federal regulations strictly govern the disclosure of information regarding patients who have been involved in a federally assisted alcohol or drug abuse program. Not only does a patient include persons enrolled but also includes any person who has applied or been interviewed for a such a program. Former and deceased patients are also protected under these regulations. In general, these treatment programs are allowed to release neither information that could identify the patient nor that the individual ever sought treatment at the facility. Information may be released only with written consent by the patient, in a medical emergency, under specified research activities, with a valid court order, or to law enforcement personnel when a patient commits a crime or threatens a crime against program personnel on the premises of the program (Brooks 1997:884–87).

When a therapist violates patient confidentiality, civil lawsuits may be brought against the clinician for breach of duty, defamation of character, or invasion of privacy. To summarize:

1. **The clinician has an obligation to keep the patient's communication private except under limited exceptions.**
2. **Special attention to the confidentiality of federally funded alcohol and drug treatment center records is mandated by law.**
3. **When the patient's mental health is the basis for a lawsuit or if the patient sues the psychiatrist, the privilege to confidentiality is waived.**
4. **The clinician should first verify with the patient and patient's attorney the legality of a subpoena requesting records prior to releasing them.**

Managed Care

Managed care organizations regulate the utilization of health care services. The advent of managed care has significantly altered the practice of inpatient psychiatry. Length of stays has shortened and hospitalization has moved to acute crisis stabilization rather than long-term treatment. Despite this dramatic shift, the expected standard of care for mental health providers has remained unchanged.

Malpractice suits against managed care organizations are restricted by the Employee Retirement Income Security Act of 1974 (ERISA). ERISA was passed by Congress in an effort to protect employees covered by self-funded plans. In self-funded plans the employer pays for employee benefits such as pensions and health care rather than purchasing an insurance policy and paying premiums. As a federal statute, ERISA preempts state law and effectively prevents those individuals covered by employee-sponsored health plans from suing for negligence claims.

A series of legal cases have begun to define the parameters of liability for managed care organizations. In 1986 the California Court of Appeals examined a managed care organization's liability regarding denial of care by reviewers in the case of *Wickline v California.* In this case a surgeon requested eight additional days for a patient to treat an occlusion of the terminal aorta following surgery. The medical reviewer granted only four days and the patient was discharged. The patient experienced complications after discharge that resulted in readmission and the amputation of her leg. The patient sued Medi-Cal. Although the jury trial ruled in her favor against Medi-Cal, the appeals court emphasized that the doctor had not appealed the reviewer's decision, and therefore Medi-Cal did not have the opportunity to participate in the decision to discharge. The court stated, however, that third-party payors can be held liable when medically inappropriate decisions result from deficits in the design or implementation of cost containment mechanisms.

In the case of *Wilson v Blue Cross of Southern California* the Blue Cross insurance company notified an inpatient psychiatric unit that they would no longer fund the inpatient stay of a man admitted for depression, anorexia, and drug dependency. The psychiatrist did not file an appeal and the patient was discharged. Less than one month later the patient committed suicide. In contrast to the Wickline case, the appellate court stated that although the physician did not appeal the decision, this did not relieve the reviewer from liability. Here both the physician and the reviewer were subject to possible liability.

Hospitals may also bear liability if clinicians are pressured to discharge patients due to lack of financial resources. In *Muse v Charter Hospital of Winston-Salem* (a non-ERISA case), a sixteen-year-old male was discharged from an inpatient psychiatric unit when his insurance benefits ended. The adolescent committed suicide approximately two weeks after discharge, and his family sued. The North Carolina Court of Appeals stated that the hospital could bear liability if they required the physician to prematurely discharge a patient when the insurance benefits ran out. The family was awarded $1 million dollars in compensatory damages and $6 million dollars in punitive damages.

These cases illustrate the importance of appealing cases when they are denied by a reviewer. Courts have also held that physicians have a duty to disclose involvement of economic issues in their treatment decisions and to continue treatment despite denial if treatment has been recommended. Managed Care Organizations (MCOs) have a duty to review with reasonable care and to select appropriate providers in delivering that care.

Currently legislative reforms regarding ERISA's limits on suing MCOs are being reviewed. **At the present time important guidelines for the physician to minimize liability with MCOs include:**

1. **Have treatment guided by the patient's need and not financial reimbursement by the insurance company.**
2. **Appeal refusals by MCOs when refusals are not medically sound.**
3. **Refer patients without financial resources to alternate care when their funding is denied rather than stopping all treatment.**
4. **Carefully review all MCO contracts for any gag clauses that prohibit the discussion of alternate treatments.**

5. **Maintain excellent documentation of appeal refusals, the reviewer's name, credentials, and the time and date of the refusal.**
6. **Consider arranging a second opinion regarding your recommended treatment from a respected colleague.** (Resnick 1997)

Minor's Rights in the Medical Setting

A **minor** is an individual who has not yet reached the legal age of majority as determined by the state. In the United States eighteen years of age represents the age of majority. In general, treatment provided to a minor requires parental consent except in emergencies. The practitioner who treats a minor absent parental consent can be liable for battery, even if there is no adverse outcome (*Zoski v Gaines* 1935). In situations in which a parent refuses necessary medical care, the physician may file medical neglect charges with the local child welfare service. A judicial hearing can be arranged on an emergency basis to determine if the parent's treatment refusal will be overridden. Following the Rehabilitation Act of 1973, Congress has passed legislation prohibiting the withholding of medical care (to include nutrition and hydration) from a handicapped infant. Lifesaving treatment must be administered unless the infant is irreversibly comatose or if the provided treatment would only prolong eventual death (Nurcombe 1994:67)

An **emancipated minor** is one for whom parents no longer have legal control but the child is still under the age of majority. Emancipation can be established by marriage, entry into the military, and independent employment and living. In general, emancipated minors are presumed competent to make decisions regarding their care.

A **mature minor** is one who though not fully emancipated possesses the developmental maturity to competently make certain medical decisions. The definition of mature minor varies according to state statute but generally requires the minor be at least fifteen years of age. Several researchers propose that children fourteen years or older have the cognitive ability to consent to medical treatment and therefore should be presumed competent. One guideline in conducting a formal competency evaluation of a minor involves assessing: (1) the child's knowledge of the disease, treatment, and prognosis; (2) educability should the child not have the requisite knowledge; (3) cognitive capacity to weigh options, risks/benefits, and consequences of choosing an option; (4) capacity for self-determination; and (5) emotional freedom (absence of a psychiatric illness or impairment) (Nurcombe and Partlett 1994:69).

A minor's right to have an abortion was addressed by the U.S. Supreme Court in the case of *Planned Parenthood of Central Missouri v*

Danforth (1976). The Supreme Court held that a pregnant minor has the right to privacy regarding the decision to have an abortion. Parental consent was not an absolute requirement for a minor to obtain an abortion. Although the court reasoned that not every minor would be competent to give effective consent to an abortion, the court provided no guidelines in the determination of competency nor whether parental notification was required. The majority of states have enacted legislation that requires some degree of parental involvement in a minor's decision making regarding abortion (Nurcombe and Partlett 1994:64–65).

Situations where the court may become involved in a minor's treatment include referrals for child abuse and neglect, an emancipated minor's refusal of treatment, and decisions related to abortion. In these instances the court can appoint a guardian *ad litem* who serves to protect the child's interests and makes recommendations to the court.

When faced with legal issues related to the treatment of minors:

1. **Determine if the minor is emancipated and can provide their own consent for treatment.**
2. **Determine if the minor is considered a mature minor by state statute and can consent for treatment.**
3. **Determine the legal guardian of the minor if the minor cannot legally consent to treatment.**
4. **Provide care in emergency situations where immediate action is necessary while attempting to notify the legal guardian.**
5. **Consider referral to child protective services if the parent or guardian refuses necessary treatment for a minor unable to give legal consent.**
6. **Discuss recommendations with the guardian *ad litem* if one has been appointed.**

Case Example Number 1

Sarah is a thirty-eight-year-old single woman treated in an outpatient psychiatric clinic for major depression. Sarah has a past history of suicide attempts that include an overdose of Xanax and an attempted hanging. Sarah's hanging attempt resulted in a psychiatric hospitalization when she was thirty-three years old. During the first week of this hospitalization Sarah denied having suicidal feelings and was taken off suicide precautions. Within twenty minutes of her change in status level, Sarah attempted to hang herself with torn sheets. After four weeks Sarah was discharged and has been followed as an outpatient on a weekly basis.

At her last outpatient psychiatric appointment, Sarah tells her psychiatrist that her boyfriend broke up with her that same day when he learned that she was diagnosed as HIV positive the week prior. Sarah is despondent and tearful. Though she denies any specific suicide plan, she refuses to sign a no-suicide contract. Sarah is voluntarily admitted to a psychiatric inpatient unit. Upon admission she is placed on a one-to-one suicidal watch. On the next day she states she has no suicidal thoughts. On day 3 she is removed from the one-to-one watch and placed on fifteen-minute checks. The managed care reviewer notifies the hospital that funding is no longer considered appropriate as there is no documentation of ongoing suicidality.

Case Analysis

1. A thorough suicide risk factor assessment should be conducted on admission and documented in Sarah's chart. Indicators for Sarah's high risk of suicidal behavior upon admission include:
   a. A previous history of suicide attempts.
   b. A past history of depression.
   c. A recent breakup with her boyfriend.
   d. Recent notification that she is HIV positive.
   e. An inability to contract not to harm herself.
   f. A tearful and despondent mood upon admission.
2. Ongoing suicide assessments should be conducted and documented in the chart. Important areas to include in these follow-up suicide assessments include:
   a. Sarah's previous psychiatric records, both inpatient and outpatient. A review of Sarah's previous psychiatric hospitalization documents Sarah's attempt to hang herself despite her statements that she was not suicidal. Although Sarah is presently denying self-harmful feelings, her past history indicates that such statements are not always reliable. The treatment team needs to weigh the risks and benefits of increasing her level of freedom. As Sarah's previous suicide attempts will remain a part of her past history, she will always be considered at a higher risk for suicidal behavior when compared with a person without such a history. It is unlikely, however, that she can be maintained on a twenty-four-hour suicide watch indefinitely. When making clinical status changes, the treatment team will need to document the reasoning for the changes to include con-

sideration of past suicide attempts. In addition, an up-to-date suicide risk assessment should be conducted and documented prior to any change.

   b. In difficult cases the clinician should consider having a second opinion consultation regarding the decision to increase the level of freedom. Should Sarah attempt to harm herself, then the physician can demonstrate that other reasonable practitioners would also have made a similar judgment call thus decreasing the potential risk of liability.
   c. The hospital should follow its own suicide prevention policies. If the suicide prevention plan specifically prohibits patients on a suicide watch from having a belt, then the hospital will likely be held liable should Sarah attempt to harm herself with her belt. By violating their own policy, no expert witness would be required to testify that the hospital fell below their own established standard of care.
3. The physician and hospital should make clinical decisions independent of authorized funding by the managed care reviewer. Should the clinician feel ongoing care is necessary, then the clinician can:
   a. Appeal any decision to deny care and document to whom the person spoke and reasons for denial.
   b. Consider obtaining a second opinion regarding the need of ongoing care.
4. Areas for potential liability in this case include:
   a. Failure to assess, diagnose, or foresee suicide risk.
   b. Failure to adequately evaluate suicide intent.
   c. Failure to adequately supervise or monitor.
   d. Failure to provide appropriate pharmacotherapy.
   e. Failure to remove potentially harmful items.
   f. Failure to obtain previous records.

Case Example Number 2

Rick is a twenty-four-year-old male who is taken to the emergency room after his wife called the police when he threatened to kill her with an AK47 assault weapon. Rick is admitted to the psychiatric unit on a seventy-two-hour hold. Rick has a previous history of physically abusing his wife. Rick is currently abusing cocaine. Previous medical records indicate Rick has been admitted previously with a diagnosis of cocaine psychosis. The urine drug screen on this admission is positive for cocaine.

When examined, Rick denies any intent to harm his wife and states that she has "blown the whole thing up." Rick reports no thoughts of harming anyone or himself. There is no evidence of psychosis. Rick meets criteria for cocaine dependence and antisocial personality disorder. Rick does not meet criteria for an affective disorder. Rick's wife calls and notifies you that he has told her that when he gets out of the hospital he plans to "pay her a visit that she will never forget." Rick reports that he made this call but only told his wife he was coming to pick up some clothes from his home. He is asking to be discharged from the hospital.

Case Analysis

1. Rick has multiple risk factors for future dangerousness, which include:
   a. Past history of violent behavior.
   b. History of ongoing cocaine abuse.
   c. Continued alleged verbal threats toward his wife.
   d. Familiarity with and access to weapons.
2. The examiner should conduct a thorough risk assessment to include:
   a. A collateral history of violence from Rick's wife.
   b. A thorough drug and alcohol history.
   c. Review of previous psychiatric and medical records.
   d. Review of any police records if available.
   e. Review of Rick's previous use of weapons and violence.
3. The examiner has the option of filing for continued civil commitment. When considering this option, the following guidelines are useful:
   a. Know your state statute regarding civil commitment. Some states allow civil commitment with a diagnosis of alcohol or drug abuse/dependence. Although all states allow civil commitment if the person has a mental illness and represents a danger to others, precise definitions regarding an overt act or specific time frame for dangerous behavior vary.
   b. In most states the need for continued hospitalization is a judicial decision. Assist the court in this decision by articulating the specific risk factors for current dangerousness should you feel further inpatient treatment is necessary.
   c. Obtain a second opinion regarding potential dangerousness. If you feel Rick does not meet continued criteria for civil com-

mitment and a second opinion agrees, then your potential liability is diminished should an adverse outcome ultimately result.

4. Learn the specific Tarasoff requirements in your state and follow them accordingly.
5. Organize and document a risk prevention plan that addresses specific risk factors for violence. For example, consider a drug treatment program for cocaine dependence, anger management for impulse control, removal of all weapons from the home, individual therapy, appropriate outpatient follow-up, monitoring once discharged, and possible pharmacotherapy.
6. Areas of potential liability in this case include:
   a. Failure to assess and document risk factors for dangerousness adequately.
   b. Failure to protect potential victims.
   c. Failure to obtain past records.
   d. Failure to treat risk factors for dangerousness adequately.

Summary

As medical and legal issues become increasingly interwoven, the administrator faces the challenge of maintaining currency on how laws govern the provision of care. **General guidelines to assist the administrator include:**

1. **Consulting with an attorney when unfamiliar legal issues arise in treating patients.**
2. **Documenting a risk benefit analysis of decision making in the chart.**
3. **Learning the state statute, case law, and legislative decisions governing medical legal issues of concern.**
4. **Appealing inappropriate denials of medical care by managed care organizations.**
5. **Obtaining a second opinion/consultation in complex cases.**

There is no single solution for every health care delivery problem. An understanding of mental health law, however, will assist the administrator in ensuring the highest quality of patient care as well as decreasing liability regarding the care provided.

GLOSSARY

Confidentiality Clinician's obligation to keep communication by a patient private

Damages Monetary compensation that the law awards to one who has been injured by the action of another

Emancipated minor A youth who is under the legal age of majority but who is no longer under legal control of their parents

ERISA Employee Retirement Income Security Act passed by Congress in 1974 to protect employees covered by self-funded plans

Guardian ad litem A person appointed by the court to protect the interests of a ward in a legal proceeding

Informed consent Consent given by a competent individual who makes a voluntary decision after provided full disclosure

Intentional torts Torts involving actions in which an individual either intends harm or knows that harm may result from his or her behavior

Mature minor An individual who has not reached the legal age of majority but who possesses the developmental maturity to make certain decisions competently

Minor An individual who has not yet reached the legal age of majority as determined by the state

Negligence Failure to exercise a degree of care that a reasonable person would exercise under the same circumstances

Parens patriae The role of the state as sovereign and guardian of persons under legal disability

Privilege The patient's right to bar the clinician from testifying about professional-obtained material in a judicial or parajudicial setting

Res ipsa loquitur Latin "the thing speaks for itself"; refers to a rule of evidence whereby negligence by the wrongdoer is established by the mere fact that the accident happened provided that (1) in the absence of negligence the harm would not have occurred and (2) the thing that caused the injury is shown to have been under the exclusive control of the alleged wrongdoer

Strict liability Liability without the need to show fault

Therapeutic privilege A clinician's withholding of information from a patient to prevent obvious harm to the patient should the information be disclosed

Tort A civil wrong

REFERENCES

Addington v Texas. 1979. 441 U.S. 418, 99 S. Ct. 1804, 60 L. Ed. 2d 323.

Appelbaum, P. D., and T. G. Gutheil. 1991. *Clinical Handbook of Psychiatry and the Law,* 2d ed. Baltimore, MD: Williams and Wilkins.

Appelbaum, P. S., and L. H. Roth. 1982. Competency to consent to research: A psychiatric overview. *Archives of General Psychiatry* 39:951–58.

Application of the President and Directors of Georgetown College, Inc. 1964. 331 F.2d 1000.

Black, H. C. 1979. *Black's Law Dictionary.* St. Paul, MN: West Publishing Co.

Bongar, B., R. W. Maris, A. L. Berman, and R. E. Litman. 1998. Outpatient standards of care and the suicidal patient. In B. Bongar et al., eds., *Risk Management with Suicidal Patients.* New York: Guilford Press.

Boumil, M. M., and C. E. Elias. 1995. *The Law of Medical Liability in a Nut Shell.* St. Paul, MN: West Publishing.

Brent, D. A., D. J. Kupfer, E. J. Bromet, and M. A. Dew. 1988. The assessment and treatment of patients at risk for suicide. In A. J. Frances and R. E. Hales, eds., *American Psychiatric Press Review of Psychiatry.* Washington, DC: American Psychiatric Press.

Brooks, M. K. 1997. Ethical and legal aspects of confidentiality. In J. H. Lowinson, P. Ruiz, R. B. Millman, and J. C. Langrod, eds., *Substance Abuse—A Comprehensive Textbook,* 3d ed. Baltimore: Williams and Wilkins.

Cantebury v Spence. 1972. 464 F2d 772, 787.

Cruzan v Director, Missouri Department of Health. 1990. U.S., 110 S. Ct. 2841.

Drane, J. F. 1985. The many faces of competency. *Hastings Center Report* 15:17–21.

Friedman, R. S. 1989. Hospital treatment of the suicidal patient. In D. G. Jacobs and H. N. Brown, eds., *Suicide: Understanding and Responding. Harvard Medical School Perspectives on Suicide.* Madison, CT: International Universities Press.

Hermann D. J. 1997. Informed consent. *Mental Health and Disability Law in a Nutshell.* St. Paul, MN: West Publishing.

Hoven v Kelble. 1977. 79 Wis. 2d 444, 256 N.W. 2d 379.

Humphrey v Cady. 1972. 405 U.S. 504, 92 S. Ct. 1048, 31 L.Ed. 2d 394.

Klassen, D., and W. A. O'Connor. 1988. A prospective study of predictors of violence in adult male mental health admissions. *Law and Human Behavior* 12:143–58.

Lipari v Sears, Roebuck and Co., and United States. 1980. 497 F. Supp. 185, D. Neb.

Litman, R. E. 1989. Hospitals and suicides: Lawsuits and standards. *Suicide and Life-Threatening Behavior* 12:212–20.

Meisel, A. 1979. The "exceptions" to the informed consent doctrine: Striking a balance between competing values in medical decision making. *Wisconsin Law Review* 2:413–88.

Meisel, A., H. L. Roth, and C. W. Lidz. 1977. Toward a model of the legal doctrine of informed consent. *American Journal of Psychiatry* 134:285–89.

Melton, G. B., J. Petrila, N. G. Poythress, and C. Slobogin. 1997. *Psychological Evaluations for the Courts—A Handbook for Mental Health Professionals and Lawyers,* 2d ed. New York: Guilford Press.

Muse v Charter Hospital of Winston-Salem, Inc. 1995. 452 SE 2nd 589, NC Ct. App.

Naidu v Laird. 1988. 539 A. 2d 1064, Sup. Ct. Del.

Natanson v Kline. 1960. 300 P.2d 1093.

Nurcombe, B., and D. V. Partlett. 1994. *Child Mental Health and the Law.* New York: Free Press.

O'Connor v Donaldson. 1975. 422 U.S. 563, 95 S. Ct. 2486, 45 L.Ed 2d 396.

Parham v J. R. 1979. 442 U.S. 584, 99 S. Ct. 2493, 61 L. Ed. 2d 101.
Peck v Counseling Service of Addison County. 1985. 499 A. 2d. 422, Sup. Ct. Vt.
Planned Parenthood of Central Missouri v Danforth. 1976. 428 U.S. 52.
Rennie v Klein. 1983. 720 F. 2d 266, 3d Cir.
Resnick, P. J. 1997. Psychiatric malpractice. Paper presented at the American Academy of Psychiatry and the Law, Board Review Course, Denver, Colorado.
Resnick, P. J., and C. L. Scott. 1997. Legal issues in treating perpetrators and victims of violence. *Psychiatric Clinics of North America* 20:473–87.
Robertson, J. D. 1988. *Psychiatric Malpractice: Liability of Mental Health Professionals.* New York: Wiley.
Rogers v Commissioner. 1982. 457 U.S. 291, 102 S. Ct. 2442, 73 L. Ed. 2d 16.
Rouse v Cameron. 1966. 373 F. 2d 451, D.C. Cir.
Schloendorff v Society of New York Hospital. 1914. 211 N.Y. 125, 105 N.E. 92, N.Y.
Schubert, F. A. 1996. *Grilliot's Introduction to Law and the Legal System,* 6th ed. Boston: Houghton Mifflin.
Simon, R. I. 1987. *Clinical Psychiatry and the Law.* Washington, DC: American Psychiatric Press.
Tarasoff v Regents of University of California. 1976. 131 Cal. Rptr. 14, 551 P.2d 334, Cal.
Vacco, Attorney General of New York v Quill. 1997. 117 S.Ct. 2293, 138 L.Ed.2d 834.
VandeCreek, L., and S. Knapp. 1983. Malpractice risks with suicidal patients. *Psychotherapy: Theory, Research, and Practice* 20:274–80.
Wack, R. C. 1993. The ongoing risk assessment in the treatment of forensic patients on conditional release status. *Psychiatric Quarterly* 64:275–93.
Washington v Glucksberg 1997. 117 S.Ct. 2258, 138 L.Ed.2d 772.
Weiner, B. A., and R. M. Wettstein. 1993. Legal issues in providing treatment. In B. A. Weiner and R. M. Wettstein, eds., *Legal Issues in Mental Health Care,* 112–13. New York: Plenum Press.
Wickline v California. 1986. 192 Cal. App. 3d 1630, 239 Cal. Rptr. 810, Cal. App. 2 Dist.
Wilson v Blue Cross of Southern California. 1990. 222 Cal. App. 3d 660, 271 Cal. Rptr. 876, Cal. App. 2 Dist.
Wyatt v Aderholt. 1974. 503 F. 2d 1305, 5th Cir.
Wyatt v Stickney. 1972. 344 F. Supp. 387, M.D. Ala.
Youngberg v Romeo. 1982. 457 U.S. 307, 102 S. Ct. 2452, 73 L. Ed. 2d 28.
Zoski v Gaines. 1935. 260 N.W. 99, Mich.

CHAPTER 6

Documentation for Health Care Administrators

Marshall B. Kapp, J.D., M.P.H., and Douglas Mossman, M.D.

Clinical record-keeping plays a key role in providing good mental health care. Mental health professionals use clinical records to refresh their memories of facts related to a particular patient's treatment. Records also can play a crucial role in helping members of a multidisciplinary team exchange information about their patients and in telling future caregivers about a patient's past symptoms and responses to treatment.

As most health care professionals are keenly aware, patient records are not merely clinical tools; they also are legal documents. Writing in the clinical record produces tangible documentation for later scrutiny of the nature and quality of mental health services delivered. A patient's clinical record may become central evidence in resolving a potentially broad range of legal issues.

Clinical records can often have a significant influence on the emotional, financial, and legal well-being of patients and providers. For example, a patient who seeks disability benefits or who sues a careless automobile driver for accident-related injuries will frequently rely on clinical records to document the presence and extent of the claimed disability or injury. Health care professionals have a legal duty to properly document patient care; if a failure to live up to this duty causes injury to a patient, individual professionals and their employing agency or facility can be held liable for the violation (*Fox v Cohen* 1980). Courts have frequently enunciated common law principles concerning the appropriateness of medical records. Patients can sue providers who fail to keep adequate records for "spoliation of evidence" (*Smith v Superior Court* 1984; Goodnight and Davis 1992), that is, for keeping records so poorly that the evidence necessary to succeed in a claim for benefits or damages is unavailable.

Besides attending to their common law legal obligations, clinicians nowadays must maintain records that meet the requirements of a variety of private agencies, third-party payers, statutes, and regulations. The Joint

Commission on Accreditation of Healthcare Organizations (JCAHO) has strict record-keeping standards, which it sets out in its accreditation manuals for acute, long-term, inpatient, and ambulatory settings. Individual agencies and facilities establish procedures by adopting internal bylaws and rules. Most states prescribe record-keeping practices in laws affecting institutions, agencies, or individual licensure. Private insurers often request extensive documentation that clinicians delivered appropriate services and that the patient's condition justified the services rendered. Additionally, federal statutes and regulations establish record-keeping requirements for patients with Medicare and Medicaid coverage, and a physician may be involuntarily terminated from these programs for records deficiencies (*Koh v Perales* 1991). Noncompliance with legal record-keeping requirements also may jeopardize licensure, JCAHO or insurance status, jobs, and staff privileges.

In this chapter we deal with several aspects of clinical record-keeping, with special attention to mental health care. We explore (a) legal and financial uses of the medical record, (b) allocation of responsibility for record-keeping, (c) practical guidelines for proper documentation of care, (d) patient access to records, and (e) confidentiality.

Legal and Financial Uses of Clinical Records

Records, Patients, and Legal Issues

Medical evidence plays a part in many kinds of civil and criminal cases. This evidence—which often consists of, or relies heavily on, clinical records—often includes information about mental health matters.

One type of legal case in which the clinical record invariably is crucial is the professional liability (malpractice) civil action. In a malpractice lawsuit a plaintiff (often a patient or relative) alleges that a health care professional (or agency or facility) deviated from acceptable standards of care (i.e., was negligent) and seeks cash compensation for injuries that directly resulted from that deviation. When attorneys consider suing for professional malpractice, they almost always have the records examined by an expert in the related field. In some states this is required. Thus, the available documentation of care may determine whether a suit even gets filed. If the patient and attorney proceed with a lawsuit, the legal outcome will depend on the records at least as much as on the actual quality of care provided, because the records will be the main source that experts use to debate whether the treatment was acceptable and the jury uses in its verdict. In a malpractice suit the written record can be the defendant-provider's greatest friend or worst foe.

Patients may file other kinds of lawsuits in which clinicians are not defendants but for which their psychiatric records will play a crucial role. Consider, for example, suits filed under the Americans With Disabilities Act of 1990, 42 U.S.C. § 12101 et seq., and § 504 of the Rehabilitation Act of 1973, 29 U.S.C. § 794, which protect persons with mental or physical disabilities from employment discrimination. If a patient-plaintiff alleges discrimination by an employer, the employer's defense may turn in part on mental health treatment records that show that the plaintiff cannot function properly on the job. Similarly, personal injury lawsuits brought because of casualty (accident) occasioned by the fault of another (e.g., an automobile crash) frequently turn on the nature of clinical proof produced.

Psychiatric records may play a critical role in legal cases in which a patient's current or past mental condition affects the law's view of his or her actions or decisions. All states allow criminal defendants to present evidence showing that, because of their mental condition, they should not be punished at all or not be punished as severely as the ordinary person. In such cases clinical records documenting past psychiatric problems may be crucial to establishing the seriousness and genuineness of their disorder. For a host of other legal tasks—standing trial, making a will, entering into a business contract, getting married, and making medical treatment decisions, to name a few—individuals must be competent, that is, they must have specific, legally defined capacities. Often, legal matters arise in which a party seeks to undo a previous decision, alleging that the individual was not competent when making the decision. For example, relatives who feel unreasonably excluded from a will sometimes challenge the validity of the document, saying when the testator made the will, delusions or dementia compromised his or her competence. In assessing such challenges, determinations about an individual's past competence may hinge on what clinical records say about the individual's thinking and behavior around the time that he or she made the decision in question.

Finally, clinical records can strongly influence a patient's legal entitlement to disability benefits. Depending on their work history, patients who become disabled by psychiatric illnesses may file claims for Social Security Disability Insurance (SSDI) or Supplemental Security Income (SSI). Patients also may request cash benefits from private disability insurance policies, workers' compensation systems, and private or public health insurance provisions.

These commonly arising types of legal cases illustrate how mental health professionals, agencies, and facilities have fiduciary duties to patients that extend beyond strictly clinical interventions, duties that include reasonable efforts to promote their patients' legal, social, emotional, and economic well-being. If, by keeping inadequate records, a clinician failed to vigorously advocate for his or her patient's legal entitlements, a court could find the clinician negligent for deviating from an acceptable standard of care. Health care providers' fiduciary duties are especially compelling when persons with mental disorders are concerned: these individuals often have the greatest need for the legal, social, emotional, and economic assistance that clinicians can offer.

Records and Financial Issues

Clinical records play crucial roles in utilization review (UR) and quality assurance (QA) programs. Third-party payment for inpatient mental health services is generally tied to a facility's having UR and QA programs that (at least attempt to) scrutinize the appropriateness, necessity, and quality of clinical care. At the initial level of review these programs function almost exclusively through examinations of clinical records to see whether they justify claimed payment for services clinicians expect to perform or have already rendered. Managed care's increasing domination of the mental health care marketplace is already pressuring service providers to produce clinical records that can pass UR and QA muster and thus support claims of cost-effective care.

Clinical records also are essential evidence in patient-provider disputes over the propriety and amount of professional fees billed. In such unfortunate circumstances the clinical record is the best means for clinicians to show exactly what care they provided and why.

When judges and juries examine and evaluate the circumstances and quality of mental health care, the tangible, material document containing the clinical record generally exerts an extremely persuasive impact on their thinking. Government and private reviewers who have health care backgrounds also give the written record great weight. As a realistic matter, the general presumption in legal review is: If it is written, then it happened; if it is not written, then it did not happen (*Abille v United States* 1980). Poor, sloppy, incomplete records invariably raise a red flag, and—fairly or unfairly—create the impression of poor, sloppy, incomplete care. Courts have held that a missing or incomplete record justifies a rebuttable presumption that the quality of care was substandard (*DeLaughter v Lawrence County Hospital* 1992).

Responsibility for Record-keeping

A facility's or agency's bylaws, policies, and procedures should identify which persons are responsible for creating and maintaining the various por-

tions of a clinical record. Thus, to meet their own policies' requirements, facilities and agencies must educate their professional staff thoroughly about their specific documentation responsibilities.

As a general operating principle, documentation should be based on the documenter's firsthand, direct knowledge about the patient. Responsibility for documentation falls on the professionals who make the observations, conduct the interview or test, or render the treatment that they are documenting. For example, notes about a prescription should be made by the physician who prescribes the drug, nursing notes by each nurse involved in patient care (Weiler 1994), consulting reports by the consultant, and so on. This principle applies in any type or size of delivery setting.

As a practical matter, the growing trend toward a treatment team approach means that almost all inpatients and many outpatients will have several different professionals contributing to their written records. This may be especially true for persons with mental disorders, who may have a variety of related and unrelated medical and nonmedical problems and who thus often receive attention from many different members of a treatment team. **When several different actors are providing and documenting patient care, agencies and facilities must compel their professionals to read regularly and carefully other team members' entries.** This obligation applies especially to psychiatrists, who usually have ultimate responsibility for key decisions about care and therefore need to stay abreast of each patient's full clinical and social picture.

Documentation duties cannot be delegated away, as, for example, from a physician to a nurse. Each professional is responsible for documenting personal observations, impressions, and actions. Although verbal orders are permissible when necessary, they must be verified shortly afterward by a written record notation. In many treatment settings individuals' record entries must receive the countersignature of a supervising or licensed professional (e.g., when the attending physician countersigns notes by medical students or physicians' assistants). In such situations the countersigning individual assumes legal responsibility for the content of that notation, and should always scrutinize (and, if necessary, amend) records before countersigning them.

Guidelines for Documentation

Ordinarily, clinical records are admissible as evidence in legal proceedings. This is because courts usually deem them to be accurate and reliable, having been made in the regular course of business (i.e., patient care) by persons with direct knowledge of the facts being documented, when those facts occurred. When records do not satisfy these conditions, courts place less reliance on them, frequently to the detriment of the professional, agency, or facility that is depending on those records to justify past conduct.

The actual form of record-keeping will vary depending on practice setting. JCAHO standards and state licensing statutes contain detailed descriptions of record-keeping requirements for hospitals, home health care agencies, and nursing facilities. Other types of health care settings have wide latitude to style their own form of record-keeping through design of internal policies and procedures. One popular form of record-keeping is the "problem-oriented" medical record, although this format has some detractors (Donnelly and Brauner 1992). **The following generic "do's and don'ts" for documentation are advisable wherever mental health care occurs.**

1. Written patient records should be accurate and truthful. If the treatment being rendered is less than satisfactory, falsifying records may only further injure the patient and the legal position of the provider. Given scientific advances in the forensic specialty of questioned document analysis and the unwillingness of modern treatment team members to cover up for their colleagues' misdeeds, any attempt to falsify a clinical record stands a good chance of being eventually discovered. Proof of such an attempt by a mental health professional could lead to federal and state prosecution for criminal fraud, licensure disciplinary action, liability insurance termination (*Mirkin v Medical Mutual Liability Insurance Society of Maryland* 1990), and civil liability to the patient for improper care or fraud (*Moskovitz v Mt. Sinai Medical Center* 1994). These adverse legal consequences are in addition to the obvious ethical problems associated with deception and dishonesty toward the patient and the public, to whom health care providers owe an obligation of fidelity (Prosser 1992).

2. Documentation of care should be thorough and complete. This does not require the production of a full-length psychiatric textbook for each patient encounter. As was stated earlier, however, legal decision makers (i.e., judges and juries) often assume that if something was not written in the clinical record, then it probably did not happen (Berner 1998). Partial record-keeping implies partial health care (*University of Texas Medical Branch at Galveston v York* 1991).

A good mental health record ought to include: identifying patient data, informed consent information, results of diagnostic tests and assessments, background and historical data, progress notes, current psychological and psychiatric evaluations, current medications, diagnoses, consultations, correspondence and phone calls, suggestions or directives, failed or canceled appointments, documentation of supervision (if any), prognoses, any releases of information by the patient, and termination notes (Moline, Williams, and Austin 1998).

3. Clinical records should be legible. Writers should use abbreviations sparingly, judiciously, and only in compliance with the facility's or agency's approved list. Sloppiness in documentation creates a presumption of sloppiness in patient care and of the mental health professional's need to hide or obscure certain facts about the patient's treatment. Additionally, considerable amounts of valuable time are lost when another member of the treatment team (usually a nurse or pharmacist) must double check the meaning of an illegible written entry or order (Kozak, Kittus, Smith, Fitzgerald, and Langfeld 1994). Worse yet, an illegible but unchecked order may result in misunderstanding and improper care (e.g., administering the wrong drug or drug dosage). For these reasons dictating record entries should be encouraged while emphasizing that the professional dictating notes should carefully read—and, if necessary, correct—the transcribed versions before signing them.

According to a 1994 report by the American Medical Association, medication errors stemming from misinterpreted physicians' prescriptions were the second most prevalent and expensive claim in 90,000 malpractice actions over a period of seven years. In 1994 the average indemnity payment for the 393 most recent medication-error claims was $120,722, with a range of $5,000 to $2.2 million (Cabral 1997).

4. Documentation must be timely. Because the professional's memory naturally fades over time, notes that are made near or at the time of the event are likely to be most accurate. The authors know about several cases in which an agency's or professional's vulnerability to a successful malpractice suit hinged on the presence or absence of a note written shortly before an unfortunate incident. Further, contemporaneous entries create a more favorable impression of overall patient care. Specific time limits for updating clinical records are established by Medicare regulations (currently fifteen days from a hospitalized patient's discharge), JCAHO standards, and internal organizational bylaws. Mental health professionals should be familiar with specifically applicable time limits, but should consider them a maximum period to be bettered whenever possible.

5. One should not overcorrect mistakes. Corrections should be obvious and legible, consisting of a single line drawn through the otherwise readable error. Writers should enter, initial, and date a change above or next to the error. White-outs, erasures, total obliterations, and destruction of complete pages create an inference of secrecy that can seriously undermine the professional's credibility, and such charting activities are highly inadvisable. An attorney, judge, or jury may interpret as destruction of relevant evidence actions that, to a mental health professional, seem like innocent attempts at neatness.

6. A patient's clinical record is no place for jousting with or editorializing about the patient, family, facility or agency, or other health care professionals (Hirsh 1998). Every entry in the record should serve a legitimate patient care purpose. Thus, appropriate notations consist of objective observations and reports and clinically significant impressions. These items should be expressed in a sober, value-neutral, nonjudgmental manner. Frustration and other feelings should be expressed in other, more appropriate fora.

Many psychodynamically oriented therapists make process notes that they keep separate from the official clinical record maintained by the facility or agency (Weiner and Wettstein 1993). Process notes do not need to be objective in the way that progress notes should be; unlike progress notes, which are used for operational and descriptive purposes, process notes are supposed to contain a therapist's speculations and fantasies. No legal rule prohibits this practice of, in essence, maintaining two sets of clinical books. Mental health professionals and administrators should realize, however, that in most jurisdictions, process notes may be "discoverable" (i.e., subject to disclosure in legal proceedings), and patients may have the same right of access to process notes as they do to official clinical records (Melton, Petrila, Poythress, and Slobogin 1997).

Records and Liability Prevention: "Writing Smart"

Once mental health professionals learn how crucial documentation is in the outcome of malpractice litigation, they may respond to fears of litigation by writing ever-more-copious progress notes. More effective than the strategy of writing more, however, is learning how to write smart. But clinicians can write smart only if they understand how the clinical record might influence legal decision-makers in a malpractice suit. Our key point is that administrators should encourage clinicians to succinctly document their thoughts and decisions at crucial points during a patient's care.

To illustrate, we consider the inpatient care of an individual admitted following a suicide attempt. Such an individual probably represents a much-higher-than-average source of liability risk for inpatient facilities: past suicide attempters are highly likely to try to harm themselves again, and hospital suicides are very likely to lead to malpractice litigation. Although persons who commit suicide seem to be the direct or "proximate" cause of their own deaths, courts often view psychiatric patients as helpless, childlike victims of their own emotional urges who need protection and control by responsible authorities (Appelbaum and Gutheil 1991; Gutheil 1984). Psychiatrists thus have been found negligent for not assessing, hospitalizing, restraining, or taking other steps to prevent suicide (Smith and Bisbing 1988). By contrast, courts that have found for defendant physicians have recognized the uncertainty of the treatment process and the patient's own responsibility for the suicide (Simon 1992).

To help potential legal fact-finders appreciate the reality of clinical uncertainty, clinical records should describe regular, frequent assessments of patients' responses to treatment and the clinicians' exercise of judgment. Mental health care involves multicausal processes. Clinical records that reflect the weighing of many factors can help courts appreciate how clinicians have used their reasonable (if imperfect) judgment (Simon 1992).

Clinicians also should record their risk-benefit judgments in progress notes. For example, before a patient who has attempted suicide receives a therapeutic pass, the psychiatrist who writes the order for the pass should also write a note explaining how the patient's condition has improved. The note should also explain that risks and benefits have been considered, and that the professional thinks the pass's benefits outweigh its risks. Documentation of such considerations would help defend the professional against charges of malpractice should that patient harm himself outside the hospital (Simon 1992).

Judgment, soberly stated reflections, and the weighing of pros and cons can all be recorded succinctly in progress notes. If malpractice litigation occurs, the professionals' judgment and unique knowledge will count for a great deal—if professionals documented their judgments and knowledge in the clinical record. We stated earlier that the record is no place for verbal battles between clinicians; it also should never reflect disparaging views of the patient being discussed. When writing progress notes, clinicians should always realize that their entries could become evidence in court; it might even help to imagine a hostile attorney reading one's entries aloud in open court (Gutheil 1980). Progress notes should not include ridicule, sarcasm, or derogatory comments that would offend a reasonable person or bias a judge or jury against the treating professionals.

Storing and Maintaining Records

Treatment facilities and agencies should physically retain clinical records in a secure storage place for as long as possible. With the aid of microfilm and microfiche technology it is easily feasible to maintain records for at least as long as the mental health professional is in practice or the health care organization is in existence. In the rare situation in which space or cost limitations make this prohibitive, agencies and facilities should retain records at least past the jurisdiction's applicable statutory minimum (in most states, around seven to ten years from the last patient contact). Medicare requires that records be kept for at least five years, 42 Code of Federal Regulations §482.24(b)(1). The statute of limitations for medical malpractice negligence actions (generally one or two years, but sometimes longer) provides no guidance in this matter. In most jurisdictions, the statute of limitations does not begin to run until the patient discovers (or should have discovered) the existence of an injury, even when discovery occurs long after the alleged substandard act or omission. **Institutions should not automatically discard patient records after an individual's death, because many legal rights that are dependent on those records may become exercisable by the patient's surviving relatives or other designated persons.**

Documenting Informed Consent

When a patient (or legal surrogate) either gives or withholds informed consent for a recommended diagnostic test or therapeutic intervention, documentation should show (1) that the legally necessary process of doctor-patient communication preceded the patient's decision, (2) that the patient acted voluntarily, and (3) that the patient was competent.[1] If the patient's written record does not sufficiently spell out these three conditions of legally effective consent or refusal, an after-the-fact reviewer might conclude that they did not obtain.

Clinicians and administrators often misunderstand the clinical and legal significance of printed consent forms for medical interventions. A consent form's value depends entirely on the degree to which it accurately reflects what really happened between doctor and patient. From both a clinical and legal perspective, written consent forms are meaningless unless the doctor did what the form says was done. The written form may assume only a subsidiary role in a clinical and legal encounter: it can memorialize the process of discussion and interaction, but should not be a substitute for that process.

Whether or not they use a separate, written consent form, mental health professionals also should document directly in the patient's chart those facts establishing the voluntary, competent, and informed nature of the consent or refusal. The advisable volume of such a note depends on the particular circumstances. Usually, a substantive but brief summary statement is sufficient. If, however, the proposed intervention is especially risky or invasive (e.g., administering clozapine or electroconvulsive therapy), it may be wise to record a more elaborate written description of the facts surrounding consent or refusal. Similarly, greater detail in the written note is advisable when the professional senses, based on prior general or specific experience, that the particular patient or family might later sue if the treatment is unsuccessful.

Some mental health professionals often ask a third party (such as a nurse) to witness consent-related conversations in the record, or have their patients read and initial chart entries. In some circumstances (e.g., interviews conducted for legal purposes), professionals will audiotape or videotape an entire evaluation or treatment procedure and include the consent process in the opening part of the recording. All these documentation practices are legally permissible. The extent to which precautions of this sort are advisable depends in part on the setting, context, and type of services rendered; it also depends on how well one tolerates legal uncertainties, as opposed to preferring to act with maximum cautiousness and legal conservatism.

Psychiatric patients frequently take many different medications and run a significant risk of adverse reactions to them. Psychiatrists and other mental health professionals must tell patients about, help them understand the risks of, and discuss reasonable alternatives to, any proposed pharmaceutical intervention. The clinical chart should reflect the details of such disclosures, and should also show how the clinicians conscientiously monitored the patient for signs of adverse drug reactions.

In 1997 the voluntary organization National Council on Patient Information and Education (NCPIE) in Washington, DC, began an implementation strategy for its "Action Plan for the Provision of Useful Prescription Medicine Information." Among other things, national education campaigns conducted by NCPIE aim to improve communication about prescription medicines. Messages are targeted to specific patient groups and health care professionals using television, radio, print, public service announcements, reports, brochures, and posters.[2]

One of the most difficult situations in the consent context arises when a patient leaves a mental health facility or agency "against medical advice" (AMA).[3] At the time of departure caregivers should diplomatically but firmly ask patients to sign a form saying that they have been told the potential adverse consequences of treatment refusal, and releasing providers from any potential legal liability related to injuries that result from treatment refusal. If the patient refuses to sign such a form, mental health professionals should report that action itself in the clinical chart, along with a description of their efforts to dissuade the patient from ending treatment AMA.

Patients' Access to Records

The paper, films, and other tangible objects constituting a patient's medical record are the legal property of the mental health facility or agency that created the record. **Institutions need never, and should never, relinquish the original versions of those items to the patient or to anyone else absent a specific court order.**

Yet, as more mental health patients demand increased participation in their clinical care, an issue has arisen concerning their right to obtain the information contained in the tangible documents. The strong and steady trend is toward a broad legal expansion of patients' rights to information contained in their records.

Patients treated today in federal health care facilities (such as those operated by the Departments of Veterans Affairs and Defense) may get access to the information in their own medical records under the authority of the Federal Privacy Act, 5 U.S.C. § 552(a). In several jurisdictions mental health care recipients in a variety of state, municipal, nonprofit, and proprietary settings now have access to their records, either as a result of judicial decisions or, in about half the states, legislation. **Mental health administrators and staff members who handle records should keep abreast of legal provisions concerning patient access to records that affect their agencies and facilities.**

They must also know about any exceptions (e.g., therapeutically privileged comments) or special procedures that their jurisdiction recognizes. One example of such a procedure is the mandatory involvement of a third-party buffer like an attorney in some states. In those states the provider must give a copy of the patient's record to the patient's attorney instead of the patient, on the theory that the attorney will exercise discretion in deciding what information to divulge to the patient. Some states allow providers to give patients a summary of the record rather than a complete copy. **Additionally, administrators must consider voluntary guidelines, such as JCAHO standards or the American Hospital Association's Patient Bill of Rights, that support broad patient access to information about one's own mental health care.** Ultimately, virtually any patient who really wants access to the clinical record can satisfy that desire through the initiation of litigation, and this empowerment will continue and expand in the coming years.

Not all clinicians approve of this trend toward granting patients enhanced access to their records. For example, some clinicians interpret record requests as expressions of mistrust or as indications that patients are assuming an adversarial posture. Though this perspective often contains more than a kernel of truth, being defensive about what is in a patient's records can be counterproductive. Letting patients see their clinical records lets them know their caregivers are comfortable with their care; often, patients come away from such experiences feeling more informed about their problems, more satisfied with their treatment, and more positive about their caregivers (McLaren 1991). In addition, granting access to information contained in the clinical record can be a way to open or facilitate a dialogue and can thereby improve the entire professional-patient relationship.

Confidentiality

Mental health professionals daily hear or read very personal, intimate information concerning persons under their care and, often, their families. This knowledge of personal patient information imposes certain duties of confidentiality on the mental health professional (Hermann 1997). **As a general precept, mental health professionals have the duty to hold in confidence all personal patient information entrusted to them,** and patients can expect them to fulfill that duty. Confidentiality obligations and their concomitant legal and ethical consequences will become ever more complex and challenging as medical records are increasingly computerized (Computer Science and Telecommunications Board, National Research Council 1997; Rind, Kohane, Szolovits et al. 1997; Sweeney 1997; Frasca 1996; Woodward 1995).

Physicians' ethical duty to keep confidences is found in sources as old as the Hippocratic Oath and as recent as the latest version of the American Medical Association's *Principles of Medical Ethics.* Confidentiality is usually part of the implicit contract between doctor and patient, in which patients expect that what they say will remain confidential. The duty also emanates from the fiduciary or trusting nature of the professional-patient relationship, that is, from the expectation that the professional will maintain confidentiality to protect the patient's interests. This broad ethical principle has been given legally enforceable status through numerous civil damage suits. In addition, most, if not all, of the state practice acts and regulations contain provisions that make violation of the duty of confidentiality a potential ground for revoking, denying, or suspending a mental health professional's license to practice.

A mental health professional's legal problems are compounded if an unauthorized disclosure is also false and injurious to a patient's reputation. In such cases, the patient could bring a civil action against the professional for the tort of defamation (libel if written, slander if spoken). Additionally, repeating a patient's false and injurious statements about a third party could also make the mental health professional legally liable to that third party. Hence, particularly with sensitive and potentially harmful information, extreme discretion is always in order.

Limits of the Confidentiality Duty

Mental health practice frequently requires professionals to consider whether other relevant factors in a particular case justify or even compel them to override their prima facie, or presumptive, obligation to maintain confidentiality (Duckworth and Kahn 1997). Although mental health professionals have a prima facie duty not to reveal information about patients, there are several recognized situations in which other duties supersede the duty of confidentiality. We list five examples of such situations here.

1. Mental health professionals may share *necessary* information with individuals who, in effect, join the treatment team, for example, with physician consultants asked to evaluate medical problems or caregivers to whom they are referring the patient for future care. Notice the emphasis in the previous sentence on the word "necessary." A psychiatrist who asks an internist to evaluate an outpatient's high blood pressure probably should tell the internist the patient's diagnosis, current medications, and other history that might affect the consultant's decision-making. Telling the internist about the patient's sexual fantasies may not be necessary, however, although such issues are central to the patient's current psychiatric care.

2. A patient may waive, or give up, the right to confidentiality, if this is done in a voluntary, competent, and informed manner. This type of waiver is accomplished daily in the mental health arena to make information available to third-party payers (i.e., insurers, Medicare or Medicaid, and managed care organizations), QA and UR auditors, and other public and private entities, including the patient's legal representative. When patients request the release and transfer of information about their treatment, mental health professionals have an affirmative obligation to cooperate fully. Failure to do so may compromise continuity and effectiveness of patient care, and could compromise patients' access to cash entitlements (e.g., SSI, SSDI, or other disability payments).

Many mental health agencies and facilities have special procedures and personnel for handling information transfer outside their institutions. Because any professional may need to make such transfers, however, all staff members should know how to obtain proper, thorough, written documentation before honoring a patient's informed, voluntary request to release information. Staff members should also verify the identity and legitimate authority of the record recipient before releasing the requested information.

Although many psychiatric patients want professionals to share information with involved family members, caregivers should never take such a desire for granted. Often, however, patients will give implicit or explicit verbal approval for sharing at least limited information about treatment. If the circumstances surrounding the treatment make such a disclosure appropriate, professionals may respect the patient's wishes and discreetly share information with family members (Petrila and Sadoff 1992).

3. Another exception to the general rule about confidentiality stems from the so-called "Tarasoff duty." This duty was first enunciated in a 1970s California case involving a patient who killed a woman named Tatiana Tarasoff. Though the duty is familiar to most mental health professionals, it often is misstated as a duty to warn. In fact, **the final Tarasoff decision (***Tarasoff v Regents of University of California* 1976**) established the principle that, when the safety of innocent third parties is in jeopardy, the general requirement of confidentiality should yield so that a psychotherapist can take reasonable steps to protect third parties from harm. Sometimes—but not invariably—taking such steps will require breaching confidentiality.**

For instance, if a patient makes a credible, serious threat to kill a specific victim, and if the patient appears intent on carrying out the threat, a therapist may have to warn the potential victim, call law enforcement officials, or take other confidentiality-breaching actions to fulfill the duty to protect. If, however, the therapist arranges for the patient to undergo hospitalization—during which time the intended victim will be safe—there might be no need to warn the victim immediately, and, if hospital treatment resulted in the patient's ceasing to intend violence toward the victim, there might never be a need to breach confidentiality at all.

Many state legislatures have passed laws specifying the types of circumstances that trigger the Tarasoff duty; in other states, Tarasoff-like court decisions have defined when the duty arises; in some states, no law or case has yet established the contours of the duty. Although there is no set of nationwide, uniform rules about what specific circumstances trigger a legal duty to breach confidentiality, most mental health professionals recognize a moral duty to protect the public from their patients' aggression. **Administrators should know what legal rules (if any) apply in their jurisdiction, and should help their professional staff learn how to comply with such rules when the need arises.**

4. The patient's expectation of confidentiality must yield when a state's laws require mental health professionals to report the existence of certain enumerated conditions in their patients to specified public health authorities. The content of mandatory reporting statutes and regulations varies somewhat among states. Thus, for example, all states require mental health professionals to report suspected child abuse, but reporting suspected cases of elder abuse or neglect is required in only 42 states; the other eight states encourage professionals (via a grant of legal immunity) to report that suspicion, but do not require reporting. Mandatory reporting requirements may be based on the state's inherent police power to protect and promote the general health, safety, and welfare of the community. They also may be based on the state's inherent *parens patriae* power to protect those who are unable to protect themselves.

5. Finally, **mental health professionals may be compelled to reveal otherwise confidential patient information by the force of legal process, that is, by a judge's court order requiring such release.** This is a possibility in any type of lawsuit in which the patient's physical or mental condition is an issue in dispute. To understand when such a release is actually mandatory, mental health professionals must understand the difference between a subpoena and a court order.

Mental health professionals may receive two types of subpoenas. A *subpoena ad testificandum* is a directive from a clerk of a court to appear at a specified time and place for the purpose of giving sworn testimony. A *subpoena duces tecum* directs one to bring certain identifiable tangible items, such as medical records, at the time of testimony. **Mental health professionals should never ignore a subpoena, but they should realize that a subpoena may be challenged legally before they actually have to comply with it and release sensitive information.**

When a mental health professional receives a subpoena (i.e., the subpoena is personally delivered to him or her), the professional should notify the concerned patient immediately. The patient, through his legal representative, may then take the opportunity to ask a judge to quash the subpoena because the requested information is protected under the state's testimonial privilege statute. If the judge agrees, the professional will not have to repeat any confidential information or disclose contents of the patient's records.

The statutory therapist-patient testimonial privilege, which is one aspect of the larger concept of confidentiality, varies substantially across jurisdictions with regard to which types of therapists and information are covered. Mental health professionals are obligated to testify only when the patient declines to challenge the subpoena or the judge rejects the challenge and orders disclosure over the patient's objection (*Rost v Board of Psychology* 1995). Noncompliance with a court order constitutes contempt of court and is criminally and/or civilly punishable.

Medical information concerning a patient's alcohol or narcotic dependency or treatment is specifically protected by federal law against unauthorized disclosure. This extra legal caution reflects a recognition of the extremely sensitive nature of this kind of information and the potentially deleterious effects of its being revealed inappropriately. Serious criminal and civil sanctions may be imposed for improper release of such information.

The entire area of medical confidentiality presently is in a state of flux (Turkington 1997). On 11 September 1997 the U.S. Department of Health and Human Services (DHHS) submitted to Congress an eighty-one-page report entitled "Confidentiality of Individually-Identifiable Health Information," calling for a national set of standards to replace—or at least supplement—the current patchwork of state and federal statutes, regulations, and judicial rulings pertaining to this subject. In the following months, this recommendation became a topic of heated debate among health care providers, users of medical information, and patient advocacy groups (Bates 1997). The 1996 Health Insurance Portability and Accountability Act (HIPAA), Public Law No. 104–191, required that DHHS take some action in terms of medical privacy by 21 February 2000 if Congress did not pass suitable legislation by 21 August 1999.

Conclusion

Information generated during relationships between mental health providers and their patients is clinically and legally important to the patients, professionals, and the institutions and agencies where those relationships take place. This importance is reflected in legal requirements concerning methods of documentation, patient access to information about themselves, and confidentiality. Clinical records are, in many ways, the stories of patients' lives. Those stories should be told accurately and should be treated with no less respect than patients themselves deserve.

NOTES

1. A discussion of the appropriateness and permissibility of coerced treatment of psychiatric patients is beyond the scope of this chapter.
2. The NCPIE web page is http://www.aoa.dhhs.gov/aoa/dir/151.html.
3. Issues surrounding involuntary commitment and retention of psychiatric patients are beyond the scope of this chapter.

GLOSSARY

Casualty Pertaining to an accident

Common law Judge-made law, based on legal precedent and relevant social values, customs, and beliefs

Competence The legal ability or capacity to engage in a specific legal activity, such as executing a will or contract

Confidentiality Health care provider's obligation not to reveal personal information about a patient to others unless the patient has given permission or another legally recognized exception applies

Defamation A civil wrong (tort) in which the wrongdoer has published to others false and damaging information about an individual

Fiduciary relationship A relationship, built on trust, in which the more powerful party (e.g., a health care provider) is obligated to act in the best interests of the less powerful party (e.g., a patient)

Malpractice Deviation from professionally acceptable standards of care, usually unintentionally (i.e., negligently)

Parens patriae Literally, "father of the land," referring to the state's inherent authority to act to protect from harm individuals who are not capable of protecting themselves

Prima facie On its face, or presumptively true, but capable of being rebutted or overturned

Privacy Act Federal statute, 5 U.S.C. Sec. 552(a), which (among other things) provides to patients being treated in federal facilities a right of access to their own medical records

Process notes Detailed notes of therapy sessions kept by some psychodynamically oriented therapists that may contain very personal information about the patient and the therapist's speculations

Progress notes Notes made in the patient's chart for operational and descriptive purposes

Spoliation of evidence A civil wrong for which a health care provider may be found liable; involves keeping patient records so poorly that the evidence necessary for a patient to succeed in his or her own claim for benefits or personal injury damages is unavailable

Statute of limitations Specific time period, set by statute within a jurisdiction, within which specific types of legal claims may be filed

Subpoena A document issued by the clerk of a court commanding the recipient to appear in a case for a specific purpose. A subpoena ad testificandum is a directive to appear at a specified time and place for the purpose of giving sworn testimony. A subpoena duces tecum directs one to bring certain identifiable tangible items, such as medical records, at the time of testimony

Tarasoff duty Mental health professional's duty, which varies among jurisdictions, to take some form of action to protect third parties from dangers posed by that professional's patient

Testimonial privilege Created by statute and varying in detail among jurisdictions, testimonial privilege gives an individual the right to prevent a witness (e.g., a mental health professional) from testifying about information obtained through a special relationship between the witness and that individual claiming the privilege

REFERENCES

Abille v United States. 1980. 482 F. Supp. 703 (N.D. Cal.).

Appelbaum, P. S., and T. G. Gutheil. 1991. *Clinical Handbook of Psychiatry and the Law,* 2d ed. New York: McGraw-Hill.

Bates, D. W. 1997. Quality, costs, privacy and electronic medical data. *Journal of Law, Medicine, and Ethics* 25:111–12.

Berner, M. 1998. Write smarter, not longer. In L. E. Lifson and R. I. Simon, eds., *The Mental Health Practitioner and the Law: A Comprehensive Handbook.* Cambridge, MA: Harvard University Press.

Cabral, J. D. Y. 1997. Poor physician penmanship. *Journal of the American Medical Association* 278:1116–17.

Computer Science and Telecommunications Board, National Research Council. 1997. *For the Record: Protecting Electronic Health Information.* Washington, DC: National Academy Press.

DeLaughter v Lawrence County Hospital. 1992. 601 So.2d 818 (Miss.).

Donnelly, W. J., and D. J. Brauner. 1992. Why SOAP is bad for the medical record. *Archives of Internal Medicine* 152:481–84.

Duckworth, K., and M. Kahn. 1997. Interface with the legal system. In A. Tasman, J. Kay, and J. A. Lieberman, eds., *Psychiatry,* vol. 2. Philadelphia: W. B. Saunders.

Fox v Cohen. 1980. 406NE2d 178 (Ill. App.).

Frasca, T. A. 1996. Issues of confidentiality in the information age. *Pharos* 59:17–19.

Goodnight, D. R., and D. R. Davis. 1992. Spoliation of evidence: The unnecessary tort. *Journal of Health and Hospital Law* 25:232–41.

Gutheil, T. G. 1980. Paranoia and progress notes: A guide to forensically informed psychiatric recordkeeping. *Hospital and Community Psychiatry* 31:479–82.

Gutheil, T. G. 1984. Malpractice liability in suicide. *Legal Aspects of Psychiatric Practice* 1:1–4.

Hermann, D. H. J. 1997. *Mental Health and Disability Law in a Nutshell.* St. Paul, MN: West Publishing.

Hirsh, H. L. 1998. Medical records. In S. S. Sanbar et al., eds., *Legal Medicine,* 4th ed. St. Louis: Mosby.

Koh v Perales. 1991. 570 NYS2d 98 (NY App. Div. 1991), appeal denied 575 NYS2d 455 (NY).

Kozak, E. A., R. S. Dittus, W. R. Smith, et al. 1994. Deciphering the physician note. *Journal of General Internal Medicine* 9:52–54.

McLaren, P. 1991. The right to know. *British Medical Journal* 303:937–38.

Melton, G. B., J. Petrila, N. G. Poythress, et al. 1997. *Psychological Evaluations for the Courts: A Handbook for Mental Health Professionals and Lawyers.* New York: Guilford Press.

Mirkin v Medical Mutual Liability Insurance Society of Maryland. 1990. 572 A.2d 1126 (Md.Ct.Special Apps.).

Moline, M. E., G. T. Williams, and K. M. Austin. 1998. *Documenting Psychotherapy: Essentials for Mental Health Practitioners.* Thousand Oaks, CA: Sage Publications.

Moskovitz v Mt. Sinai Medical Center. 1994. 69 Ohio St.3d 638 (Ohio Supreme Ct.).

Petrila, J. P., and R. L. Sadoff. 1992. Confidentiality and the family as caregiver. *Hospital and Community Psychiatry* 34:136–39.

Prosser, R. L. 1992. Alteration of medical records submitted for medicolegal review. *Journal of the American Medical Association* 267:2630–31.

Rind, D. M., I. S. Kohane, P. Szolovits, et al. 1997. Maintaining the confidentiality of medical records shared over the Internet and the World Wide Web. *Annals of Internal Medicine* 127:138–41.

Rost v Board of Psychology. 1995. 659 A.2d 626 (Pa.).

Simon, R. I. 1992. *Clinical Psychiatry and the Law,* 2d ed. Washington, DC: American Psychiatric Press.

Smith v Superior Court for City of Los Angeles. 1984. 198 Cal. Retr. 829 (Cal. App.).

Smith, J., and S. Bisbing. 1988. *Suicide: Caselaw Summary and Analysis.* Potomac, MD: Legal Medicine Press.

Sweeney, L. 1997. Weaving technology and policy together to maintain confidentiality. *Journal of Law, Medicine, and Ethics* 25:98–110.

Tarasoff v Regents of University of California. 1976. 551 P.2d334 (Cal. Supreme Ct.).

Turkington, R. C. 1997. Medical record confidentiality: Law, scientific research, and data collection in the information age. *Journal of Law, Medicine, and Ethics* 25:113–29.

University of Texas Medical Branch at Galveston v York. 1991. 808 SW2d 106 (Tex.Ct. App.).

Weiler, K. 1994. Legal aspects of nursing documentation for the Alzheimer's patient. *Journal of Gerontological Nursing* 20:31–40.

Weiner, B. A., and R. M. Wettstein. 1993. *Legal Issues in Mental Health Care.* New York: Plenum Press.

Woodward, B. 1995. The computer-based patient record and confidentiality. *New England Journal of Medicine* 333:1419–22.

CHAPTER 7

Financial Management

Ray G. Newman, Ph.D.

In this chapter we will examine three areas of financial management that will provide assistance in contending with certain financial administrative matters. The first area is the relationships within financial statements to develop a basis not only for assessing an organization but also for comparisons of one set of financial statements to another. Second, we will look at budget considerations that deal with break-even analysis. Break-even analysis uses the relationships among cost, volume, and pricing to determine a point at which there is neither profit nor loss. This technique can be used as well to factor in a desired profit. Costs are utilized according to their nature, that is, fixed or variable. Finally, we will consider key financial ratios. For an organization these are analogous to vital signs that physicians use when assessing a patient's health. Managers of organizations do the same thing. We look at key vital signs, interpret the results, and consider managing and changing them for improvement.

Financial Statements

There are several primary financial statements with which you may already be familiar. An audited set of financial statements, whether for your organization or someone else's, will contain at least a balance sheet, an income statement, and a statement of cash flows. Each of these is reviewed here to determine its underlying nature. The connections between and among the statements will be identified to show how they relate. Initially, however, a few of the underlying accounting concepts will be discussed to help put later sections in perspective.

Double-Entry Accounting

There are certain fundamental principles in accounting that accountants follow, and they are based today, as they have been for about five hundred years, on **double-entry accounting.** The double-entry bookkeeping technique actually dates back to 1494 to a Franciscan Monk named Fra Luca Pacioli. It was he who invented double-entry accounting, and it has been with us ever since. So accountants have a long-term tradition behind this concept.

From this accounting convention came **debits** and **credits.** These are words and devices to ensure there are exactly as many dollars on the debit side of the ledger as on the credit side. That is why accountants are obsessive about "balancing the books" and making sure the debits equal the credits. The words have little meaning in and of themselves; they are merely terms of convenience to facilitate recording transactions and maintaining equality between the two.

Accrual and Cash Bases of Accounting

You may have heard references to the accrual versus the cash basis of accounting. What is the difference? The concept of **accrual accounting** refers to recording and matching revenues and expenses in the period in which they are either earned or incurred, irrespective of when cash is received or disbursed. Regardless of when cash actually changes hands, these events, or transactions, are recorded to provide a more accurate reflection of the financial status of the organization. The presence of accrual accounting is evident when the balance sheet includes items such as accounts receivable or accounts payable. An event or transaction can have an impact on the organization and its financial statements without an immediate effect on cash. A simple example is shown by professional services being provided to a patient in one month but whose insurance company does not pay the fee until the following month. The organization has earned the revenue and has a claim or right to receive payment for its services but has to wait to be paid. Accrual accounting records the revenue at the time it was earned irrespective of when payment is actually made. Under **cash accounting** revenue is not recognized or recorded until cash is received. Conversely, expenses are not recognized until paid.

Balance Sheet

The **balance sheet** is a snapshot of a particular moment in time that shows total assets owned by the organization, claims (liabilities) against those assets, and the residual value or equity of the owners. This structure is memorialized in the accounting equation: assets = liabilities + owner's equity. For reference only, assets (those things we own) carry a normal debit balance and are increased with a debit entry (and decreased with a credit entry). Liabilities and owner's equity have a normal credit balance and are increased with a credit entry (and decreased with a debit entry). Thus, with double-entry accounting (each transaction being recorded with equal debits and credits) the accounting equation is satisfied with equality. Having equal debits and credits does not mean transactions were recorded correctly to the proper accounts, it only means that at least the books balance.

Business Cycle

The normal cycle of business that is captured in the accounting records follows a general cycle. The owners invest in productive assets that allow them to produce the goods or services they are in business to sell. Acquiring the assets is accomplished through borrowing funds, buying on credit (these two constitute using "other people's money"), or paying cash. When the goods or services are sold, the business recognizes revenue. From this the costs of doing business are deducted. If an excess of revenues over expenses results, there is a profit; if not, there will be a loss.

A central tenet is inherent in the cycle. We invest in assets with the objective of having those assets generate revenues and therefore profits. As we realize profits, we invest in more assets to generate more revenues to produce more profits and so on. Generally, you should not invest in assets unless they are expected to maintain or increase returns (profits).

At the same time as assets are generating revenues, expenses are being incurred as part of the productive process. Employees have to be hired and paid, supplies and materiel from vendors must be on hand, plus many other operating activities that result in expenses and liabilities being incurred. If services are provided on credit and a delay occurs before cash is received, accounts receivable are created. For a hospital this is usually the single largest current asset on the balance sheet and requires constant management.

Assets

The left side of the balance sheet (table 1) shows what the organization has acquired (e.g., inventories, plant, property, and equipment) or has a right to receive as future benefits (e.g., accounts receivable). **Assets** can be tangible or intangible (e.g., goodwill, patents) that are listed in order of liquidity (ease of converting to cash). Thus, cash is shown first with longer-term assets shown further down the listing. **Current assets** are those items that are expected to be used or consumed within an operating cycle or a year, whichever is longer. For example, inventory and supplies are used in the business within a few weeks or months. **Long-term assets** such as plant, property, and equipment have useful lives extending well beyond a single operating cycle and benefit two or more accounting periods.

Liabilities

Liabilities reflect claims of outsiders against the assets of the firm. These claims can be secured, unsecured, senior subordinated, or other categories. These characteristics become important in the event of bankruptcy or liquidation. **Current** and **long-term liabilities** share the same temporal aspects as their counterparts on the asset side of the balance sheet.

Owner's Equity

This section represents the owner's claim to residual assets (i.e., what is left over after creditors' claims are considered). This equity section does not indicate market value but is based upon historical values that seldom correspond with the market valuation. This will be pursued further in a later section.

TABLE 1. Connecticut Yankee Hospital Balance Sheet as of 30 September 19xx (in thousands of dollars)

Assets		Liabilities	
Current assets		Current liabilities	
Cash and securities	10,830	Accounts payable	30,825
Accounts and receivables	40,196	Interest payable	1,778
Inventories	3,456	Current portion	
Current assets	54,482	of long-term debt	2,370
		Current liabilities	34,973
Due from affiliates	355	Self-insurance liability	19,819
Assets—limited use	59,945	Long-term debt	91,979
Plant, property, and equipment	155,514	Other liabilities	17,435
Less accumulated depreciation	59,335	Total liabilities	164,206
Net PP&E			
		Fund balances	50,361
Other	3,306	Total liabilities	
		and fund balances	214,567
Total assets	214,567		

Owner's equity is increased or decreased by investments, profits, and losses generated by the operations of the organization or by dividends distributed. The owner's equity ("fund balance" for not-for-profit organizations) in general, and retained earnings in particular, show the aggregate profit (or loss) since the day the present organization began business. It could be for one year or fifty years. The accounting equation can be seen in play on the balance sheet. Look at the totals on the bottom of the balance sheet. Total assets are $214 million, and the total of liabilities ($164 million) plus equity ($50 million) also equals $214 million.

The organization receives supplies from vendors who have a claim against the assets of the company until paid. Other claimants include bondholders (if debt is issued), employees (for earned but unpaid wages), governmental agencies (for unpaid payroll taxes and income taxes), banks (for loans), and so forth. The right-hand side of the balance sheet reflects the creditors that have claims against the assets. Anything left over is the owner's equity. (This not dissimilar to your owning a house. For example, you have invested in the house, which is the asset. The mortgage against it is a claim by the mortgagor. Any value beyond the claim against it is your equity.) Assets are listed in sequence of liquidity, and the same principle is followed on the right-hand side for liabilities. Liabilities are listed in order of debts due the soonest, such as accounts payable, usually due within thirty days. Long-term debt is anything that is due more than a year from the balance sheet date.

The fund balance reflects the cumulative profits and losses for the organization since the day it opened; not just for the current year. We will see from the income statement how the net income or loss flows into the fund balance. As long as the fund balance is positive, results of operations have been favorable; if it is negative, that is not a good sign.

Limitations

There are limitations of the balance sheet relating to at least three items: receivables, inventories, and accumulated depreciation. Operations of two identical organizations can be precisely the same but net income can be different. The discussion that follows reveals how that can happen.

Historical Costs

The basis for recording transactions is historical cost whether it was done yesterday or twenty years ago. Historical cost is the most objective and measurable method by which to value transactions or events occurring in the life of the organization. Therefore, the balance sheet does not represent today's market value of the company. For example, if you bought a building in the heart of midtown Manhattan twenty years ago for $10 million, no doubt it would be worth much more today, say $40 million. On the balance sheet the value would be shown at the original cost less depreciation (which equals **net book value;** the net book value becomes smaller each year, while the market value can continue increasing). There can be a large gap between the market value of an asset and how it is valued on the balance sheet.

Generally accepted accounting principles (GAAP) direct accountants how to record transactions and the numbers that go into the financial statement. You cannot, however, pick up financial statements from two seemingly identical companies and compare them directly expecting the same results because there are areas where alternative ways of presenting information are possible. These areas are reviewed briefly.

Accounts Receivable

Accounts receivables represent the right to receive payment for goods/services provided on credit. As you know, not everyone pays their debts. Companies have **bad debts** when customers do not pay. Uncollectibles, in part, will be a result of how extensive credit is allowed in the business. Uncollectibles reduce the gross receivables to a net realizable value, which is the amount shown on the balance sheet. Estimating how many accounts will be uncollected in the future depends on many variables. One company may declare all accounts over 150 days of age will be uncollectible, while another may use 120 days or 180 days or base the estimate on a percentage of different aging categories. Bad debt expenses on the income statement will be different, profit will be different, and this will affect net receivables accordingly.

Inventory

Inventories are recorded at cost as acquired over time. But, when they are sold, accountants are allowed to use one of several methods to account for the cost of the inventory moving out. An important point here is that the cost flow is not the same as the physical flow of the products. The physical flow in and out of the organization has no bearing on how inventory is valued on the books (except in case of the specific identification method).

You may have heard of FIFO or LIFO, which are alternative methods of valuing inventories and with the cost flow of moving inventory off the balance sheet as they are consumed in the business. **FIFO** means first in–first out. This method of inventory moves the oldest costs (not necessarily the item) out of the asset account first. In a period of generally increasing prices, the more recently acquired inventory will be at a higher cost. An organization using FIFO moves the lowest and oldest costs to the expense portion of the income statement and leaves the higher and more current costs on the balance sheet, which increases the total assets.

If using **LIFO** (last in–first out), the more recently acquired inventory cost moves off the balance sheet first, which puts more current (higher) costs to the income statement, which decreases net inventory. LIFO leaves lower inventory costs on the balance sheet, which decreases the total assets (compared to FIFO). Companies can manipulate net profit by using one method over another. Many firms desire to minimize income taxes they pay and will adopt LIFO to decrease net inventory, and therefore taxes. The weighted average method falls in between FIFO and LIFO.

Depreciation

Depreciation reflects an organization's estimate of how long its buildings or equipment will last. These assets benefit more than one accounting period and are used in the production of goods and services. Consequently, their costs are allocated over an estimated useful life and are captured as depreciation expense. One method of allocating costs is the straight-line depreciation technique, which provides an even allocation of cost over each year of estimated life. Accelerated depreciation methods result in more depreciation being charged to operations in the earlier years of its life and less in the later years. In the early years the income statement then has more expense, lower income, and fewer taxes.

Income Statement

Another key financial statement is the **income statement,** which shows revenues, expenses, and profit (see table 2). Connecticut Yankee Hospital has earned $220.8 million in revenues, incurred $218.0 million in expenses, and recognized $1.6 million in non-operating revenues, leaving a profit of $4.4 million. The difference between operating expenses and operating revenues is operating income. In this case $2.8 million. ("Operating" revenue and expenses are relative to the core business for which the organization is created. Income/expenses outside that core may be captured in "nonoperational income/expenses.") This facility has other nonoperating income, which for most hospitals derives from interest income on investments or endowments. The $4 million net profit will find its way into owner's equity (or fund balance) and increase net book value of the organization by this amount.

The income statement is presented for a particular period of time, usually a year. Remember, the balance sheet is as of a specific date (the snapshot). The balance sheet is a picture of how things stand at a particular instance in time, because a second later, it is changing due to transactions continuing to occur. The income statement is more like a moving picture because it shows what has happened over the course of a year.

Cash Flow Statement

Although most health care organizations are required to report on an accrual basis (to get that "more accurate" picture), actual cash flow is extremely important. To ignore cash is to do so at your own peril. Therefore, a company converts its accrual-based financial statements into a cash flow statement to measure actual changes in cash for the year. The third major financial statement is a **statement of cash flows** (table 3), which shows how cash was increased and decreased or how it was used and where it came from. The statement of cash flow reflects cash activities from three primary categories: operational, financial, and investment activities. Operational cash flow is mostly from the income statement—cash flows from running the day-to-day operations of the company. Investing cash flows reflect the activity of investing in assets such as equipment. Financial cash flows reveal activities in financing the company, for example, issuing debt.

The beginning point of the statement of cash flows is the "bottom line" of the income statement (prepared on the accrual basis). One might

TABLE 2. Connecticut Yankee Hospital Statement of Revenues and Expenses for Year Ended 30 September 19xx (in thousands of dollars)

Patient revenues (net)	220,864
Operating expenses	
Salaries and benefits	133,958
Supplies	59,239
Depreciation	10,056
Interest	4,768
Bad debts	9,999
Total expenses	218,020
Operating income	2,844
Non-operating revenue (expenses)	1,572
Excess of revenues over expenses	4,416

TABLE 3. Connecticut Yankee Hospital Statement of Cash Flows for Year Ended 30 September 19xx (in thousands of dollars)

Cash flow from operating activities	
Income from operations	2,844
Adjustments to reconcile net income to net cash	
Depreciation	10,363
Increase in other liabilities	3,854
Increase in self-insurance liabilities	1,329
Decrease in other assets	1,124
Decrease in payables/accruals	(278)
Increase in receivables	(308)
Restricted fund transfers	(895)
Net cash provided by operations	18,033
Cash flow from investing activities	
Non-operating revenues (expenses)	1,572
Restricted gifts	793
Use of restricted fund transfers	231
Restricted fund investment income	129
Transfers to affiliates	(573)
Increase in limited assets	(2,463)
Increase in insurance agents	(2,925)
Increase in tax-exempt bond funds	(12,218)
Capital expenditures	(17,162)
Net cash used in investing	(32,616)
Cash flow from financing activities	
Net incremental borrowings	18,653
Principal payments on long-term debt	(2,240)
Increase in deferred financing	(737)
Net cash provided by financing	15,676
Net increase in cash and equivalents	1,093
Cash and equivalents, beginning of year	9,737
Cash and equivalents, end of year	10,830

consider this amount to be the net amount of cash to ultimately flow in from operations; however, we need to measure actual cash from operations for the year in addition to capturing cash flows not reflected on the income statement.

When we convert from the accrual to the cash basis, we begin with the ending figure on the income statement and add back noncash activities such as depreciation (table 3). In addition, without going into great detail, changes are measured in current assets and current liabilities (the short-term components of the balance sheet) during the year. As an example, services can be rendered to a patient this year but not be paid for until a future period. Although the revenue is increased and shown on the income statement, cash is not received; therefore, an increase in accounts receivable results, which means less cash was actually collected during the year. Conversely, if accounts receivable decreases during the year, more cash was brought in and reflects an increase in cash flow for the year. Other current assets are interpreted in the same manner.

When shifting from an analysis of current assets to current liabilities, the impact is just the opposite. If accounts payable increases, that means our trade creditors are in effect providing financing for the organization. This is interpreted as a source of cash and increased cash flow from operations. By the same token, a decrease in liabilities means we have paid off some debts and this is a use of funds (a decrease in cash flow from operations).

Noncash items from the income statement coupled with the changes in current assets and current liabilities result in the net cash provided by operations. This is why the income statement (table 2) shows less than $3 million net income but actual cash flows of $18 million were generated from operations (table 3).

The next two sections, investing and financing, correspond to the long-term activities of the balance sheet. For example, investing in equipment and other assets will result in changes in the balances on the balance sheet for fixed assets or long-term assets. Investing in assets is a use of cash that reduces the cash flow for the year.

We may have generated a positive $18 million this year from operations, but the company used $32 million in investing activities; on the other hand, the organization received a net $15 million in inflows from financing sources. The net result from the three areas is a $1 million positive increase in cash for the year. That amount, when added to the cash balance at the end of the prior year, results in the ending cash balance for the current year. You will see that the cash account balance on the balance sheet (table 1) corresponds with the resulting cash and equivalents balance in table 3.

The statement of cash flows and its three primary activity centers have to be monitored and analyzed over time. If there is a consistent negative net cash flow year after year, then the organization is slowly consuming itself and heading for rough times. How long that takes depends in part on the amount of cash reserves available to the company. One must look at the underlying areas to determine what needs to be corrected if this situation exists.

Behavior of Costs

One of the underlying aspects of corporations is behavior of their costs. There are two categories: fixed costs and variable costs. An example will show the impact that fixed costs have on pricing, because as one moves more into a competitive environment, there can be more and more concern about whether we can price ourselves competitively. Look first at **fixed costs** as they relate to volume (see table 4). Fixed costs are those costs that do not vary with volume increases. With a volume of 100 units and fixed costs (e.g., depreciation, core staffing level of personnel, rental payments) of $10,000, the average fixed cost at a volume of 100 is of course $100. If we increase the volume to 200, fixed costs stay the same ($10,000) because they are fixed; however, the average fixed cost now drops in half to $50. If the volume increases to 300, the fixed costs still remain at $10,000, but average fixed costs will be $33. At 400 units in volume, average fixed cost decreases further to $25. The fundamental behavior of fixed costs, and the advantage gained with volume, is that if a company can increase its volume, it can spread fixed costs over that increased volume and lower the average cost. This impacts directly with the ability to set lower prices and, other things being equal, to become more price competitive.

Now look at **variable costs** (table 5). Total variable costs change as volume changes; however, variable costs per unit remain the same. For example, if an X-ray procedure requires two sheets of X-ray film each time the procedure is performed and no film is used when the procedure is not done, total costs will vary as volume changes. If we are again at 100 units (say, X-rays) and the average variable cost per procedure is, say, $10, then

TABLE 4. Fixed Costs, Volume, and Average Fixed Costs

Number of Exams	Total Fixed Costs ($)	Average Fixed Costs ($)
100	10,000	100
200	10,000	50
300	10,000	33
400	10,000	25

at a volume of 100, the total variable cost is $1,000. As volume increases, the total variable cost per unit remains the same ($10), but the total variable cost increases. At a volume of 400 procedures, total variable costs are $4,000.

Now, combine fixed costs and variable costs and see what happens in total (table 6). At a volume of 100 units, there are $10,000 of fixed costs and $1,000 of variable costs ($10 × 100), for a total cost at a volume of 100 of $11,000. This produces an average cost of $110. If the volume is increased, total costs will go up, but the average cost will come down. This is why volume is so important. If we can take part of our competitors' shares of the market place, fixed costs can be spread over more units, with lower pricing possible. For example, if we operate at a volume of 200 with the average total cost of $60, and our competitor is able to operate at an average total cost of, say $50, he can price lower than we can. But, if we can increase our volume so the fixed costs are spread over more volume, and reduce our average total costs to, say $43, then we are in a competitive position to underprice the competition and take market share away. The key feature of the behavior of costs is that fixed costs, and not variable costs, are what impact average total cost.

Break-Even Analysis

The analysis that follows briefly describes the relationships among three variables: cost, profit, and volume. These three variables can be used to

TABLE 5. Variable Costs, Volume, and Total Variable Costs

Number of Exams	Variable Costs ($)	Total Variable Costs ($)
100	10,000	1,000
200	10,000	2,000
300	10,000	3,000
400	10,000	4,000

TABLE 6. Total Fixed and Variable Costs

Number of Exams	Total Costs ($)	Average Costs ($)
100	11,000	110
200	12,000	60
300	13,000	43
400	14,000	35

calculate a break-even point. **Break-even analysis** is a quantitative tool, but before you can use this technique, you have to be able to segregate costs between fixed and variable. It is difficult to do in some types of organizations, but there are techniques for estimating portions of costs between the fixed and variable portions. Break-even analysis is a tool that tells us what level of volume we have to have just to break even; that is, to have zero profit, neither profit nor loss. This can be applied to the institution as a whole, to departments, and to sections, as long as there are units of measurement that can be used.

The basic equation (table 7) shows that total revenue equals total costs ($TR = TC$). When revenues equal costs, profits equal zero. Drilling down into the formula shows total revenue is made up of two components: the quantity of the units produced and the price we charge ($TR = Q \times P_u$). Total costs (TC) are composed of fixed costs and total variable costs ($TC = FC + TVC$). Total fixed costs are of course fixed, but total variable costs are also a function of quantity and input price or cost per unit ($TVC = Q \times VC_u$). Thus, $Q(P_u) = FC + Q(VC_u)$.

By manipulating the formula, the volume needed to break even can be determined by dividing the fixed costs by the difference between the price per unit and the variable cost per unit (table 7). Notice fixed costs are total dollars (in our example, \$10,000). The price charged and variable cost are per unit, not total. This translates into \$10,000 of fixed costs divided by the price per unit, say, \$20, less the variable cost per unit (\$10) (table 8). We can "proof" the answer by using the results to calculate the profit (see table 9). Remember, only three elements are needed to calculate a break-even point: fixed costs, price per unit and variable cost per unit.

TABLE 7. Break-Even Formula

Break-even (BE) occurs when:

Total Revenues (TR) = Total Costs (TC); where
TR = Quantity (Q) × Price per unit (P_u) and
TC = Fixed Costs (FC) + Total Variable Costs (TVC), and
TVC = Quantity (Q) × Variable Cost per unit (VC_u); therefore,
$Q(P_u) = FC + Q(VC_u)$

Restate the formula to solve for Q (break-even volume):

$BE \text{ (or } Q) = FC \div (P_u - VC_u)$

Extension of Break-Even Formula

The formula can be used also to solve for any one of components in the equation. For example, let us say the organization's capacity is such that it can sell only up to 1,000 units. If it wants to break even, and knows what the variable cost is per unit, it can determine maximum allowable fixed costs for rent, equipment, etc. Substitute the known quantities in the equation and solve for fixed costs. The 1,000 units is Q (break-even volume), the price (P_u), is the competitive price that can be achieved (say, \$20), and the variable cost (VC_u) is \$10. Solve for fixed costs. This will tell you the maximum amount of fixed costs that you can absorb and not incur a loss. Conversely, if you know your fixed costs and variable cost and you know you can sell a thousand units, then the formula can be used to solve for the price to charge to break even. The break-even formula is simplest to use when dealing in a single product/service environment.

The health care industry, like others, has many different products/services that a single organization provides. Each service may have different amounts of variable costs and reimbursement rates. Consider Diagnostic Related Groups (DRGs). We will look at a three-DRG environment. Even though DRGs can have different reimbursement rates and different

TABLE 8. Break-Even Example

Fixed Costs (FC) = \$10,000
Price per unit (P_u) = \$20
Variable Cost per unit (VC_u) = \$10

$$
\begin{aligned}
BE &= FC \div (P_u - VC_u) \\
&= 10{,}000 \div (20 - 10) \\
&= 10{,}000 \div 10 \\
BE &= 1{,}000
\end{aligned}
$$

TABLE 9. Proof of Break-Even Formula (using "income statement" format)

Revenues (1,000 × \$20)	\$20,000
Less Variable Costs (1,000 × \$10)	10,000
Equals "Contribution Margin"	10,000
Less Fixed Costs	10,000
Equals "Profit"	0

costs associated with them, we can still use the break-even formula, but we have to develop averages to use in the formula.

In the three-DRG environment we will assume there are three products (see table 10). The first product comprises 25 percent of the business volume. The organization receives $500 reimbursement for each service. Program specific fixed costs are $50,000, and the variable cost to produce this product is $300. The second product constitutes 35 percent of the business at a reimbursement rate of $2,000, has $100,000 fixed program costs, and $1,200 variable costs. The third product constitutes the other 40 percent of the business with its appropriate revenues and costs. Each has different rates of reimbursement, different fixed costs, and different variable costs. Which numbers are used in the formula? We use a weighted average calculated as shown in table 11.

The proportion of each service is cross-multiplied by the dollar amount to derive the portion of the average total contributed by each DRG. The average price of $1,225 becomes our "price per unit" for the break-even formula. A variable cost is calculated in the same manner (table 12). We have now derived a $1,225 average price, $815 for the average variable cost, and the fixed costs as stated total $750,000. Solving the equation for the break-even volume in this example shows the firm needs 1,830 units (say, admissions) to just break even (table 13). The answer can be proofed to show it is correct.

We can also modify the formula to allow for profit. Few organizations want to just break even, because they need some excess revenues over

TABLE 10. Three-DRG Example

DRG	Percentage of Volume	Rate of Reimbursement ($)	DRG Program's Fixed Costs ($)	Variable Costs ($)
1	25	500	500,000	300
2	35	2,000	100,000	1,200
3	40	1,000	150,000	800
	100		750,000	

TABLE 11. Calculation of Weighted Price for DRG Example

DRG	Percentage		Rate ($)		Weighted Revenue
1	25	×	500	=	125
2	35	×	2,000	=	700
3	40	×	1,000	=	400
			Weighted Price	=	1,225

expenses to reinvest in the company, to replace equipment, and build up and invest in other assets and so forth. If a company desires a stated amount of profit, say $50,000, then it is treated as an added fixed cost. The contribution margin, the difference between the price and the variable costs, is used to cover not only fixed costs, but the desired profit (see table 14).

We have gone from 1,830 admissions to 1,952 because the extra volume is needed to cover the $50,000 profit. This can also be proofed in the same manner as before.

For-profit organizations can also allow for necessary taxes in calculating break-even at a given level of profit. This is done by grossing up the profit figure by dividing profit by one minus the tax rate (see table 15). For example, if the tax rate is 40 percent, divide the profit by 0.6 (1 – 0.4). The company can pay taxes and still end up with $50,000 profit. As before, this means additional volume is needed to cover the cost of taxes. Now 2,033 units, rather than 1,952, are required.

TABLE 12. Calculation of Weighted Variable Cost for DRG Example

DRG	Percentage		Variable Costs ($)		Weighted Variable Costs
1	25	×	300	=	75
2	35	×	1,200	=	420
3	40	×	1,000	=	320
			Weighted Variable Cost	=	815

TABLE 13. Break-Even Calculation for DRG Example

$BE = FC \div (P_u - VC_u)$
$= 750{,}000 \div (1{,}225 - 815)$
$= 750{,}000 \div 410$
$BE = 1{,}829.27 \sim 1{,}830$ units

Proof of Break-Even Calculation for DRG Example

Revenues (1,830 × 1,225)	$2,241,750
Less Variable Costs (1,830 × 815)	1,491,450
Equals "Contribution Margin"	750,300
Less Fixed Costs	750,000
Equals "Profit"	300[a]

[a]Does not equal zero due to rounding of units.

A further variation can be applied in that, rather than a stated amount of profit, say the board wants the profit to represent 10 percent of revenue, that is, a return on sales of 10 percent versus a fixed profit amount. The same formula again is used but modified slightly. If a 10 percent profit is desired, adjust the denominator rather than the numerator. Therefore, continuing with the original example, a return on sales per unit of 10 percent equals \$122.50 (\$1,225 × 0.10). This is treated as an added variable cost. Solving the equation (table 16) shows 2,609 units are needed to produce a profit that is 10 percent of sales (see table 16 for the proof). If

TABLE 14. Break-Even Point plus Stated \$50,000 Profit

$BE = (FC + Stated\ Profit) \div (P_u - VC_u)$
$= (750{,}000 + 50{,}000) \div (1{,}225 - 815)$
$= 800{,}000 \div 410$
$= 1{,}951.22 \sim 1{,}952$ units

Proof of Break-Even Calculation plus Profit

Revenues (1,952 × 1,225)	\$2,391,200
Less Variable Costs (1,952 × 815)	1,590,880
Equals "Contribution Margin"	800,320
Less Fixed Costs	750,000
Equals "Profit"	50,320[a]

[a]Does not equal exactly \$50,000 due to rounding of units.

TABLE 15. Break-Even Point plus Stated \$50,000 Profit Net of Taxes

$BE = [FC + Stated\ Profit / (1 - \text{Tax Rate})] \div (P_u - VC_u)$
$= [750{,}000 + 50{,}000 / 1 - 0.4)] \div (1{,}225 - 815)$
$= (750{,}000 + 83{,}333) \div 410$
$= 2{,}032.52 \sim 2{,}033$ units

Proof of Break-Even Calculation plus Profit Net of Taxes

Revenues (2,033 × 1,225)	\$2,490,425
Less Variable Costs (2,033 × 815)	1,656,895
Equals "Contribution Margin"	833,530
Less Fixed Costs	750,000
Taxable Income	83,530
Less Taxes (40 percent)	33,412
Equals "Profit"	50,118[a]

[a]Does not equal exactly \$50,000 due to rounding of units.

taxes need to be factored in, follow the same procedure as before. Gross up the desired profit ($122.50 per unit) by dividing it by 1–Tax Rate.

Financial Ratios

Financial ratio analysis is used in financial management to assess how healthy the organization is. The analogy of doing this with an organization is the same as a physician or nurse diagnosing a patient. When a physician looks at vital signs of a patient, he or she cannot make a diagnosis based upon a single vital sign. For example, you cannot look at only blood pressure or temperature or only the respiration rate. A collection of indicators and statistics has to be considered to get an overall assessment of the health of a patient. Having done that, one can prescribe a regimen or a prescription for what needs to be done for the patient.

The same thing is done with organizations. Financial ratios provide the diagnostic tool for a manager as vital signs do for a physician. A major analogy to keep in mind: just as the body is kept alive by blood circulating through its system, so too an organization has to have a similar circulation to remain viable—it is called cash flow. If the blood flow for the patient is shut off, the patient dies. The same applies to an organization.

Financial ratios are the "vital signs" for organizations. They help measure the health of the organization through ratios (such as return on investments), tell how well management is doing, and provide other important indicators of management. Financial analysis is used also to determine credit risks. Outside creditors or third parties are very interested

TABLE 16. Break-Even Calculation for Profit Margin of 10 percent for DRG Example

$BE = FC \div (P_u - VC_u - Profit\ Margin)$
$= 750{,}000 \div [1{,}225 - 815 - (1{,}225 \times .10)]$
$= 750{,}000 \div (410 - 122.50)$
$BE = 2{,}608.70 \sim 2{,}609$ units

Proof of Break-Even Calculation for DRG Example

Revenues (2,609 × 1,225)	$3,196,025
Less Variable Costs (2,609 × 815)	2,126,335
Equals "Contribution Margin"	1,069,690
Less Fixed Costs	750,000
Equals "Profit"	319,690[a]

Note: 10 percent of Revenues = $319,603

[a]Does not equal exactly 10 percent due to rounding of units.

in assessing the organization's risks before lending money to the organization.

Trends of the organization's financial health are useful to determine if the status is becoming better or worse. The best measure of comparison of financial ratios is to compare them with the organization's own benchmarks. The past history for the past two or three years of the organization can be viewed to see which way trends are going. Some of the vital signs may be becoming better, some may be becoming worse. You can also compare the organization with other similar-type organizations, beyond that, and can compare to industry averages (see table 17). The sequence shown is in descending order of relevancy or adequacy of comparison. Let us take industry average. Say I am at a 1,500-bed, major teaching hospital in Manhattan. To compare the results for my institution with the industry average of all hospitals would be virtually meaningless. The average hospital in the United States is about 160 beds in size, is nonteaching, and is a community hospital. The industry average does not have much in common with my organization. So the farther away one moves from specific likenesses, or the broader the comparison base, the less accuracy there is in comparing myself to the comparison group. If I compare myself with other major teaching hospitals in New England, then the revenue is a little better. It would be even more so if I compared myself with other major teaching hospitals in New York City. The closer we get to "home," or to our specific type of operation, the more relevant the comparison is.

Here we will review some of the more common and important financial ratios. Major categories of ratios that will be reviewed are liquidity, profitability, asset management, and capital structure ratios. Liquidity ratios answer the fundamental question of whether we are able to meet short-term obligations. The current asset and current liability sections in the balance sheet are used for this purpose. Liquidity is a measure of short-term rather than long-term solvency. It indicates our relative capacity to pay our creditors, vendors, and other short-term obligations.

Three ratios of liquidity analysis are presented: current ratio, acid test, and days cash on hand. They are quite simple. You will see the numbers in the example on the balance sheet (table 1). The **current ratio** reflects our ability to cover current liabilities. It is measured by dividing current

TABLE 17. Financial Ratio Comparison Bases

Own organization benchmarks (budgeted results)	More relevant
Own organization trends (past 2–3 years)	to
Other similar groups	
Industry averages	Less relevant

assets by current liabilities. Refer to the balance sheet to locate these amounts.

Current assets ($54.5 million), on the left-hand side of the balance sheet, divided by current liabilities ($30.8 million), on the right-hand side, results in a ratio of 1.6. This says we have $1.60 in current assets for each dollar of current liability that exists today. That is, we have more than enough to cover short-term obligations. The industry average is about 2.0. Almost all industries look at a minimum of 2.0 as a heuristic rule of thumb. So the higher the ratio, the better. If the ratio drops to less than 1.0, for example, 0.75, meaning there is only 75 cents to cover every dollar of short-term debt, you are technically insolvent. That does not mean you go to jail or go to bankruptcy court immediately. But it is certainly an indication that you need to make some quick cures to turn the situation around.

The **acid test ratio** is a more severe version of the current ratio. The difference is that inventories are removed from the equation. We remove inventories because they tend to be the least liquid of current assets. Current assets typically consist of cash, receivables, marketable securities, and inventory. Inventory can be converted to cash less easily than the other current assets.

In this case, the ratio is 1.56, or $1.56 of quick assets for each dollar of short-term liability. The industry average is about 1.8, so in this example we are still slightly below. The acid test ratio will always be lower than the current ratio if inventories are present. Table 18 provides a summary listing of ratio formulas, calculations, industry average, and comparison of the sample hospital with the average.

The **number of days cash on hand** is a very interesting number because it tells us, if cash stopped coming in as of today, how long we would be able to cover operating expenses. It is the maximum safety period if cash no longer arrives. We look at the really liquid assets, cash and marketable securities ($10.8 million). Divide this figure by the average daily operating expenses derived from the income statement (table 2). Exclude depreciation because it is not a cash expense. Take the operating expenses on the income statement ($218.0 million), subtract depreciation ($10.1 million), divide the total by 365 (days in a year) and the average is $570,000 per day. The result tells us we have 19 days of cash on hand if the cash flow stopped.

Profitability Ratios

Profitability ratios are probably better known than other ratios to most everybody. These ratios tell us how well the organization is doing from a

TABLE 18. Summary of Financial Ratios

Ratio	Formula	Calculation	Hospital Ratio	Industry Average	Comparison
		Liquidity Ratios			
Current ratio	Current assets / Current liabilities	54,482 / 34,973	1.6	2.0	Negative
Acid test	Current assets—inventories / Current liabilities	54,482 – 3,456 / 34,973	1.5	1.8	Negative
Days cash on hand	Cash and marketable securities / Average daily expense	10,830 / (218,020 – 10,056) / 365	19.0	19.6	Negative
		Profitability Ratios			
Profit margin	Net income / Revenues	4,416 / 220,864	.020	.049	Negative
Operating margin	Operating income / Revenues	2,844 / 220,864	.013	.022	Negative
Return on assets	Net income / Total assets	4,416 / 214,567	.021	.039	Negative
Return on equity	Net income / Fund balance	4,416 / 50,366	.088	.077	Positive
Basic earning power	EBIT / Total assets	2,844 + 4,768 / 214,567	.036	.034	Positive
		Debt Management Ratios			
Debt ratio	Total debt / Total assets	164,206 / 214,567	.765	.488	Negative
Times interest earned	EBIT / Interest expense	4,416 + 4,768 / 4,768	1.9	3.1	Negative
Fixed charge coverage	EBIT + Fixed charges / Fixed charges	4,416 + 4,768 + 1,368 / 4,768 + 1,368 + 2,240	1.3	1.4	Negative

		Activity Management Ratios			
Inventory turnover	Revenues / Inventory	220,864 / 3,456	63.9	34.5	Positive
Current asset turnover	Revenues / Current assets	220,864 / 54,482	4.1	3.3	Positive
Fixed asset turnover	Revenues / Fixed assets	220,864 / 96,179	2.3	1.5	Positive
Total asset turnover	Revenues / Total assets	220,864 / 214,567	1.03	.79	Positive
Average collection period	Accounts receivable / Average daily revenue	40,196 / 220,864/365	66	77	Positive
Average payment period	Accounts payable / Average purchases	30,825 / 59,239/365	190	58	Negative
		Other Ratios			
Average age of plant	Accumulated depreciation / Depreciation expense	59,335 / 10,056	5.9	7.5	Positive
Price/Earnings	Price per market share / Earnings per share	28.50 / 2.21	13	15	Negative
Market/Book	Price per market share / Book value per share	28.50 / 25.18	1.13	2.1	Negative

profit perspective. They look at the revenues, how well expenses are kept under control, and how well the organization is doing in terms of profitability. These show the combined effects of liquidity, asset management, and debt on operations. Creditors are concerned with solvency and liquidity; they know profitable firms are more likely to pay off debts. We will look at five profitability ratios that creditors, banks, and stockholders are interested in. The five are: profit margin, operating margin, return on assets, return on equity, and basic earning power.

The **profit margin** ratio is a basic, fundamental measurement of profitability, one that most companies and investors look at. Profit margin compares net income with revenues. Net income is the bottom line on the income statement ($4.4 million in table 2) divided by revenues ($220.1 million). This results in a 2 percent return on sales. That is, for every dollar of revenue generated, two cents is retained as profit or the amount of revenue remaining after expenses. The industry at this time was about 5 percent. So this organization is below average for this ratio.

The **operating margin** is a subset of the profit margin just calculated. Here we look at only operating income (or income generated from those activities that we are primarily in business to conduct). Exclude non-operating revenues and expenses, normally shown near the bottom of the income statement. Operating income is not the bottom line but is the $2.8 million (table 2), which is operating revenues less operating expenses. Thus, operating income divided by operating revenues produces a 1.3 percent return compared to an industry average of 2.2. This organization generates less return on the primary business than the industry as a whole. The operating margin will be lower than the profit margin unless non-operating revenues are negative.

Basic earning power (BEP) looks at the fundamental ability of the organization to generate profits. It excludes taxes, interest, and non-operating revenues/expenses. Operating earnings before interest and taxes (EBIT) can be derived from the income statement if it is not specifically shown as a separate subtotal. In our example, add back interest expense ($4.7 million) to operating income (no taxes are involved in this example). That gives us $7.6 million. Divide by total assets ($214.5 million). This relationship shows the ability of the firm's assets to generate operating income. In this case, it is 3.6 percent. Industry average is 3.4 percent. That is, for every dollar in assets, the company produces 3.6 cents in operating earnings (before paying interest to creditors and taxes to the government) and is slightly better than the industry average.

Why do we look at total assets in this ratio? To begin with, answer the basic question of why we invest in assets (buildings, equipment, X-ray machines, or offices). We invest in assets in order to generate additional revenue. By increasing revenues, we hope to increase profits. If we invest in assets that do not have the potential of maintaining or increasing revenues and profits, then we are investing in the wrong things. The reason for investing in assets is to increase the size of the business through generation of revenues and profits. This is a way of looking at the productivity of the assets and how well they are being utilized or managed to generate profit.

Return on assets is probably a phrase most people have heard. It is similar to the BEP we just reviewed but compares the net income (rather than EBIT) to total assets. It shows the effectiveness of total assets in producing profit. It looks at the totality of the organization and the profit generated after paying interest on debt and taxes. Net income of $4.4 million (table 2) divided by total assets of $214.5 million (table 1) results in a 2.1 percent return, with an industry average of almost double that. So, per dollar of assets, the organization is not generating as much profit as the industry average.

The next ratio, **return on equity** (ROE), should be a term familiar to most individuals. If you personally have invested in bonds or stocks, by putting in, say $1,000, you measure that investment by how much you are getting back either through interest payments or the growth of stock. That is exactly what the return on equity ratio is. It is the return on equity that has been provided by owners or investors. It is calculated by dividing net income ($4.4) by equity (or the fund balance for not-for-profit organizations). In this case ROE is 8.8 percent. The industry average is a little less than that. So in this vital sign the company is doing better than the industry average. This ratio is used by investors and owners to compare to alternative investments, either on the stock market or someplace else that might generate higher returns. If a potential investor sees he or she can earn 8.8 percent by investing in the organization, compared to 10 or 15 percent elsewhere, where do you think that investor's money will go? An investor will act in a way to maximize return.

Debt Management

Now let us shift to debt management. If there is debt on the balance sheet, then we are "leveraged" because we leverage the business by using other people's money. If the firm earns more on investments financed with borrowed funds than is paid in interest costs, the return on owner's capital is magnified (leveraged). If we can generate profits by using other people's money, keeping our equity investment the same, then if profits go up, what happens to our return on equity? It goes up because a higher net income divided by the same level of total assets produces a higher return on equity. Debt management ratios are a longer-term perspective, in contrast to the liquidity ratio factors that measure short-term solvency.

Now consider the balance sheet (table 1). On the left side are the assets, the things we invest in. The things we own or invest in are financed by the right-hand side (other people's money and owners' money). People often ask how an organization is financed. Well, it is through a combination of debt and equity (those items on the right-hand side of the balance sheet), which represent the financial structure of the organization. The relative size of the debt to equity has a lot do with the ratios that come into play. We will look at three ratios in this area: debt ratio, times-interest-earned (TIE), and the fixed charge coverage.

The **debt ratio** simply says what proportion of our financing is done by debt. Look at total debt ($164.2 million) on the balance sheet. Divide the total debt by total assets. This shows 76 percent of our assets are financed with debt. The complement, of course, is that 24 percent is financed with equity. The industry average in this case is much lower (about a two-to-one ratio, or 48 percent of assets financed by debt). This firm is more highly leveraged than the average.

Having just looked at debt, we need to consider interest costs on that debt. If we have bank borrowings or long-term bonds outstanding, interest has to be paid. Interest is a fixed charge. No matter whether business is good or bad, debt obligations have to be met. So creditors are very interested in how well the organization is generating profit to cover that interest.

The **times interest earned** (TIE) coverage is a measure of how much profit is being generated to meet interest on outstanding debt. It measures the firm's ability to meet annual interest payments. The key figure is earnings before interest and taxes (EBIT) defined as before. We want to see how much profit is available before interest to cover the interest charges. From the income statement take net profit, which is $4.4 million, and add back interest expense ($4.7 million). That shows we have about $9.2 million to cover interest payments. This gives a two-to-one TIE ratio, or two times the amount of interest payments. Another way to view this is as a margin of safety that shows how much profits can fall off before we are in danger of defaulting on loans.

Many bond covenants associated with long-term debt issues set floors below which the TIE cannot go; if it dips below that threshold the organization is in violation of the bond covenants. If not cured quickly, then all sorts of nasty things can happen. The final action may be that outsiders can come in and take over the organization.

The **fixed charge coverage ratio** is an extension of the TIE ratio. The fixed charged coverage looks at all fixed charges. Interest expense is just one of the fixed charges that have to be met. There can also be lease payments, rental payments, and other types of fixed charges. In our example we have interest expense, lease payments, and the principal on the debt that we have to pay ($8.7 million). (When we have debt, we have to pay not only interest but also principal; the term debt service includes interest and principal payments.) Again, we look at how much profit is available for payments on fixed commitments. (Not all fixed charges will be shown on the financial statements. You will identify fixed charges by reviewing additional records or information in the organization.) The resulting figure is 1.3, which means we have $1.30 available to cover each dollar of fixed payments. That is a relatively thin margin of safety.

Activity Ratios

We now consider activity ratios. These are designed to indicate how well assets are being utilized and are working for us. We will look at four ratios. In these formulas, the numerator is always revenue. The four items are components of assets that are compared to revenues to see how well the assets, in part or in total, are generating revenues for us.

The **inventory turnover** (how many times during the year we sell the value of the inventory) is an indicator of the efficiency of managing inventories; the lower the turnover rate, the longer inventories are being held, which ties up cash. Inventories of $3.4 million divided by revenues of $220.8 million equal 63.9. In our example we turn inventory over 63.9 times a year, which is about once every six days. Stated another way, the value of the inventory is sold about once a week. Items included in the value of inventories shown on the balance sheet vary among organizations. Included can be pharmaceuticals on the floors and the central pharmacy, central supply, laundry supplies, plus others. Some places will inventory maybe only some of those and not others. The lack of consistency or uniformity will make comparisons with other organizations more difficult.

Now let us look at other asset categories. Revenues divided by current assets results in a **current asset activity ratio,** which means we are generating $4.20 of revenue for each dollar of current assets. Large dollar items that we invest in, such as buildings, property, and equipment, are fixed assets. These assets are designed to provide capacity and ability to generate revenues. Divide revenues by fixed assets ($214.5 million), and the resulting **fixed asset activity ratio,** shows we generate $1.03 of revenue for each dollar of fixed asset. The higher this number, the more efficient we are utilizing assets.

In the **accounts receivable ratio** the average collection period is a very important one, especially for hospitals. Accounts receivables usually is the largest single current asset for a hospital. It is one thing to extend credit and have a large amount of revenues recorded, but, if that revenue is sitting in a receivable balance rather than being collected as cash, then you do not have the cash to invest in more assets to generate more revenues (or pay your vendors or employee payroll).

The longer revenues sit in receivables, the harder it is to collect them. The older they become, the more bad debt expense incurred. Management of receivables is a critical day-to-day management tool that needs to be monitored. The accounts receivable ratio is often referred to as "days in AR." This measures how many days of revenue are outstanding. It is simply taking the accounts receivable balance ($40.2 million) from the balance sheet (table 1) and dividing by the average daily revenue. Average daily revenue is calculated by dividing the revenue for the period (in this case $220.8 million, one year's revenue) by the number of days in the period (here 365).

We have an average of a little over two months' (66 days) worth of revenue sitting in receivables. That is about average for the hospital industry. The number depends upon not only management but also on the mix of payers making up the composition of receivables. Each major category of payer (Blue Cross, Medicare, etc.) can be measured by using each with its own set of revenues and outstanding balance to see if and where delays are occurring. The business officer probably should be spending more time on a day-to-day basis in this area than on anything else.

Another activity ratio is **average payment period.** This looks at how long how it takes on average to pay vendors. In this example, we owe vendors about six months of payments. The industry average is probably closer to a month or two. Most vendors send invoices and expect payment in thirty days. Any balance due vendors means they are helping to finance the organization. Any undue habitual delay in payment to vendors can result, at some point in time, in vendors increasing prices to make up for the loss in use of cash. They can also charge interest, start delivering on a COD basis, or stop selling to the organization altogether.

The **price earnings ratio** is a market perspective of how well the prospective earnings are for the company. If you want to consider investing in a company, you do it on the basis of the profits generated by that company, both historically and what you think the profits will be in the future. If you think the profits are going to go down, you do not invest. With an average market price that the public is paying for a share of stock of $28.50, and the company generating $2.20 earnings per share, divide earnings into the market price to get a ratio of 13. This means the market is willing to pay 13 times the earnings per share to own a share in the company. Review the *Wall Street Journal* to see the range of price earning ratios that are in the marketplace. The national price-to-earnings ratio is an average of about 15. The average investor is willing to pay 15 times what the company is earning per share. If you see a stock being traded with a price earning ratio of 20, that says the market is willing to pay more than average for a share of that company's stock. Why? Because the market expects the earnings to be better than average in that company. Of course, it could be overvalued, too. The adverse is true as well. If a stock is trading at seven times earnings, the market may say that it is not producing very good profits, and so it is not as willing to pay as much for a share of it. But, by the same token, maybe it is currently undervalued, and it may take off soon.

Summary

List all of your financial ratios on a sheet of paper to obtain an overall assessment of the health of an organization. From the list can be seen where the problems and strengths are. Just as you would analyze and assess the vital signs of a patient, so too you can gauge the health of an organization. From this a corrective regimen can be prescribed as necessary.

GLOSSARY

Accounts receivable ratio Efficiency measure of management of accounts receivable; indicates how long it takes on average to collect an account; also known as days in receivables

Accounts receivables A general ledger account presented on the balance sheet that shows how much patients or payers owe the institution due to the extension of credit; a major current asset for hospitals

Accrual accounting The basis of accounting that records revenue when earned and expenses when incurred regardless of when cash is exchanged; see *Cash accounting*

Acid test ratio A liquidity measure of ability to cover short-term liabilities; determined by dividing current assets (less inventories) by current liabilities

Assets Items owned by an enterprise; can be tangible or intangible; includes items such as accounts receivable the enterprise has a right or claim to receive; categories include current assets and long-term, or fixed, assets

Average payment period Average length of time it takes a firm to pay its creditors; determined by dividing accounts payable balance by the average daily purchases on credit

Bad debts An income statement expense item reflecting the estimated uncollectible amounts in accounts receivable due to nonpayment by patients or others

Balance sheet A major financial statement that shows, for a particular point in time, the balances of assets, liabilities, and equity for a firm

Basic earning power ratio A ratio that measures the efficiency of assets to generate income (before interest expense and taxes); determined by dividing earnings before interest and taxes (EBIT) by total assets

Break-even analysis A technique to calculate a point of sales volume in which neither a profit nor a loss occurs; uses the relationship of fixed costs, variable costs, and price

Cash accounting A basis of accounting that records revenues and expenses when cash is exchanged rather than when earned or incurred; see *Accrual accounting*

Credit An accounting device to record increases in liabilities, equity, or revenue and decreases in assets; see *Debit*

Current asset activity ratio Measures the efficiency of current assets in generating revenues; determined by dividing revenues by current assets

Current assets Assets owned by the enterprise that are expected to be used or consumed within an operating cycle or one year, whichever is longer; includes cash, marketable securities, accounts receivable, inventories

Current liabilities Liabilities owed by the enterprise that are due for payment within an operating cycle or one year, whichever is longer; includes accounts payable, accrued payroll, current portion of long-term debt

Current ratio A liquidity measure of the ability of the enterprise to meet its short-term obligations; determined by dividing current assets by current liabilities

Debit An accounting device to record increases in assets and expenses, and decreases in liabilities and equity; see *Credit*

Debt ratio A ratio that reflects how much of the enterprise is financed by debt; determined by dividing total liabilities by total assets; the complement to the debt ratio shows how much of the enterprise is financed by equity

Depreciation An allocation of acquisition cost of an asset over the estimated useful life of the asset; appears on the income statement as depreciation expense and on the balance sheet as accumulated depreciation

Double-entry accounting A five hundred-year-old system accountants use to maintain equality of debits and credits in recording transactions or events in the life of an enterprise

FIFO First in–first out; an inventory valuation method to determine the value of inventories to place on the balance sheet; this method moves the older costs off the balance sheet first, leaving the more recent costs on; refers to the movement of costs rather than the physical movement of inventory items

Financial ratio analysis An analytical review of the relationships of an enterprise's accounts; used to determine the financial health of an organization by reviewing "vital signs"; categories of ratios include liquidity, profitability, debt management, activity

Fixed asset activity ratio An efficiency measure of fixed assets to generate revenues; determined by dividing revenues by fixed assets

Fixed charge coverage ratio A measure of the firm's ability to generate earnings to cover fixed charges such as interest, principle on debt, leases; reflects a margin of safety on how much earnings could drop and still cover fixed charges

Fixed costs Costs that do not vary with changes in volume; applicable to a relevant range of production; includes items such as core staffing, leases

Fund balance Represents the equity portion of the balance sheet for not-for-profit organizations

Income statement A major financial statement of the summary of revenues and expenses for an enterprise for a particular period of time; the difference between revenues and expenses represent net income (or net loss) or excess of revenues over expenses (or excess of expenses over revenues)

Inventories A current asset category representing materiel used in the production of goods or services

Inventory turnover An activity ratio representing how many times the inventory is "turned over" during the period; an efficiency measure in the management of inventory

Liabilities Debts and obligations owed by an enterprise; shown on the balance sheet using categories of current and long-term liabilities

LIFO Last in–first out; an inventory valuation method to determine the value of inventories to place on the balance sheet; this method moves the newer costs off the balance sheet first, leaving the older costs on; refers to the movement of costs rather than the physical movement of inventory items

Long-term assets Assets that are expected to benefit the enterprise over a period of two years or more; assets, other than land, subject to depreciation, amortization, depletion

Long-term liabilities Debts and obligations that are due more than one year in the future; shown on the balance sheet

Net book value Reflects the net value of an item; shown on a historical cost basis; for example, (1) net book value of an item of equipment is the difference of its acquisition cost and its associated accumulated depreciation; as the item becomes older and the depreciation accumulates, net book value declines; (2) net book value of the enterprise is the difference between total assets and total liabilities; the value can be positive or negative

Numbers of days cash on hand ratio A liquidity measure of the amount of cash on hand to meet expenses if no more cash were to be received; determined by dividing available cash (cash and marketable securities) by the average daily expenses

Operating margin ratio A profitability measure that compares operating profit to revenues; determined by dividing operating income by revenues

Owner's equity The difference between total assets and total liabilities; represents the owners' residual value in the enterprise; shown on the balance sheet; referred to as fund balance for not-for-profit organizations; see *Fund balance*

Price earnings ratio A market measure of the current and expected profitability of an enterprise; determined by dividing the market price of a share of stock by the earnings per share of the enterprise

Profit margin ratio A profitability measure; compares net income to revenues generated; determined by dividing net income by revenues

Return on assets ratio A profitability measure of the use of assets in the enterprise; determined by dividing net income by total assets

Return on equity ratio A profitability measure of the net income compared to owner's equity; determined by dividing net income by owner's equity

Statement of cash flows A major financial statement that shows the sources and uses of cash during the period; components include cash flows from operations, financing activity, and investing activities

Times interest earned ratio A debt management ratio showing earnings generated before interest and taxes (EBIT) to cover interest expense; reflects a margin of safety of how much earnings could drop and still cover interest expense

Variable costs Costs that vary with changes in volume; the relationship between variable costs and volume is a linear relationship; variable cost per unit is constant, while total variable costs increase proportionately with volume

CHAPTER 8

Managing Organization Behavior

Birge D. Reichard, Ph.D.

Understanding and managing human behavior in work organizations requires specific knowledge and focus on that task. The knowledge required comes from many disciplines—psychiatry, psychology, sociology, and business, to name a few. Organization behavior is multidisciplinary and requires one to think across boundaries as well as within them. Focus refers to the ongoing need to systematically apply the learning and not simply react by instinct or habit. Managing organization behavior requires many of the same skills required by clinicians—getting educated and trained in the requisite knowledge areas and applying that knowledge in systematic ways that are guided by principles. Concentration, observation, analysis, and working with a plan in mind are the instincts or habits of effective organization managers.

This chapter is intended to equip you with the knowledge and examples of systematic ways to apply the knowledge to enable you to work effectively and confidently in the managerial part of your role. The literature on organization behavior keeps growing as the importance of this subject in achieving organizational effectiveness continues to be relearned. Principles will be discussed here more than procedures, since each organization is unique. Examples of the application of the principles will be provided in order to stimulate your thinking about the best way to proceed in your particular organization. The citations used in this chapter deliberately include classical references that remain timeless along with contemporary sources.

The Organizational Context

Kurt Lewin (1969), often referred to as the father of applied behavioral science, was fond of saying, "There is nothing so practical as a good theory." One of his theories is expressed as a formula:

$$B = f(p.e.).$$

Translated, the formula reads that behavior (B) is a function (f) of the interaction of the person (p) and the environment (e). Because the individual is so tangible and visible, most managers, and many clinicians, interpret organization behavior on the basis of diagnosing and analyzing the individual who is acting out the behavior. This is done even when the manager or clinician knows better. It is the environment or context that so often gives meaning to the behavior. Dr. Larney Gump put it this way:

> To say, "he took off all his clothes," would have very little meaning unless one knew the context or environment in which the action occurred, such as, "in the privacy of his bedroom," "in the middle of a busy street," or "as a stroke victim learning to care for himself again." (1983:5)

The environment or context of an organization with which the individual interacts contains variables like task, purpose or direction, structure, rewards, technology, leadership, and organization culture, which profoundly influence individual behavior. The same individual interacting within different variables will behave differently. Since understanding individuals is assumed here to be an area of expertise with the target audience of this book, that is, psychiatrists, clinical psychologists, LCSW's, psychiatric nurses, etc., our focus here will be on learning about some of the important organizational variables that constitute the context, or environment (e), in Lewin's formula.

What Is an Organization?

Just as there are many ways to define an individual or a group, there are many ways to define an organization. The approach chosen here is to provide a model of an organization—its component parts—and use that to describe the variables (or the context) that must be managed in order to manage organization behavior. While there are many other models, including later ones (see Burke 1992), this one is selected because of its simplicity and ease of use. The model selected for the purpose of this book is one developed by Marvin Weisbord (1978). His book, cited in the references here, is a good tool for managers who wish to pursue this subject and organization diagnosis in more depth and with guided, practical application.

The **Purposes** box is appropriately labeled number 1. To understand any work system—at any level of the system: individual, group, or organi-

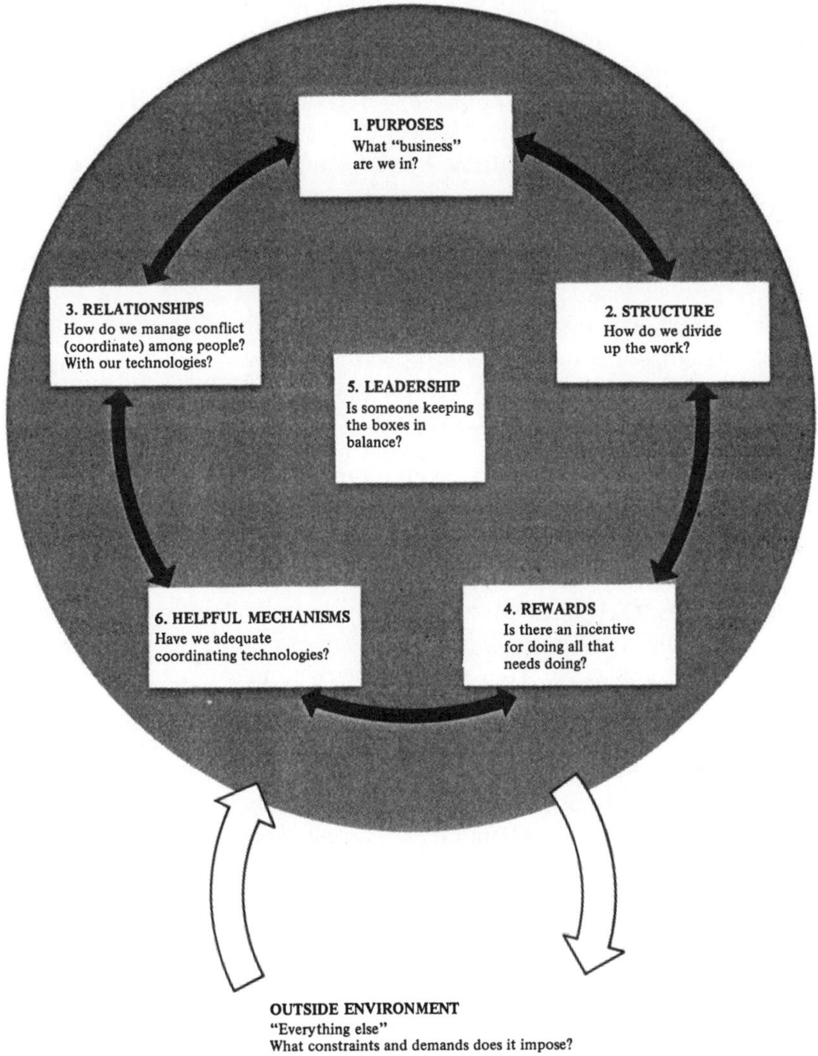

Fig. 1.Weisbord's six box model. (From Weisbord 1978, 9.)

zation—one must understand its purpose. Why is it here? to do what? for whom? At the largest system level this would be the mission of the organization. A modification of this model is extension of this box to include smaller units of the organization—or levels of the system and refer to this box as Direction Setting. Achievement of organization and group purpose is dependent upon having defined goals. At the individual level we have objectives. In all cases it is essential that people know the direction in which the organization or group is headed, and the aim of collaborative effort. One definition of a work group is people collaborating on a task. If the purpose or task is unclear or if members of the group have different understandings of them, confusion and counterproductive behavior will occur. Progress in the task will be difficult and conflict will be rife. In such an event, if the manager focuses on the individual, the intervention will be targeted on interpersonal relationships, motivation, cooperation or conflict management. The real problem here, however, is lack of clarity about what the group is convened to do. Clarifying that will resolve many of the behavior problems.

In addition to clarifying the mission or purpose, key operating goals—what must occur if the mission is to be accomplished—must be established by each work unit. Only at that time will individuals have the necessary context to think about what they can do to ensure the accomplishment of unit goals. They are then ready to negotiate objectives with their bosses. This is part of **performance management** discussed in chapter 9, "Human Resources in Mental Health Care Organizations."

Direction Setting at all organization levels, from purpose or mission (what business are we in?) to strategic organizational or system level goals, to unit goals, to individual objectives—is one of the most important tasks of management. It is probably best to assume the direction setting is not clear enough and always needs reiteration, monitoring, and reinforcement. This is especially true in today's turbulent operating environment, where things like goals and objectives are dynamic and, by necessity, are changing during an operating period.

In practice, the manager of a unit large enough to define a mission (e.g., a hospital, separate clinic, or major operational unit) must ensure that all of the key subordinate managers understand and agree upon the raison d'être of the organization. Understanding and agreement is best achieved by participation in the process of defining the mission. The rest of the management cadre must be educated to the mission, preferably by having personal, face-to-face discussion and dialogue with the key managers who created the mission.

Consider the following situation that illustrates the conflicts that arise from unclear purpose. Remember that purpose relates to what is done, for whom, and how.

A large urban teaching hospital established an Emergency Psychiatric Service (EPS) center as a satellite unit in the community. The hospital management viewed the purpose or mission of the new center as a vehicle for providing time-limited mental health services to a population that was unable or unwilling to use other forms of psychiatric treatment. The intent was to assist in the resolution of crises and/or refer to suitable resources such as community mental health centers and other community-based programs. The limited number of psychiatrists was to be used for diagnosis and consultation with other professional staff (primarily psychologists, nurses, and social workers), who were to provide brief therapy and manage referrals, family involvement, etc. The manager of the service was a psychiatrist whose career had been in private practice, was near retirement, and was recruited for the job by the hospital's chief of psychiatry, who was an old friend.

The hospital management assumed the recruit knew how to manage and did not want to offend by insisting upon an extensive orientation. The perception of the community was that a new treatment center had opened in their neighborhood. Many nonemergency clients came through the door, and the manager's background was in providing treatment. Transition care was not fully anticipated, and staff, feeling guilty about not having suitable referrals, engaged in traditional treatment. The unit became swamped and perpetuated the community view of its purpose as a treatment center. Hospital residents assigned to the unit to learn about diagnosis and consultation spent most of their time as therapists. The unit was in competition with the existing programs in the hospital and performed poorly because it was not resourced for that work. The manager constantly argued with the hospital administrator about resourcing.

This scenario could have been avoided or minimized by paying more attention to purpose. Involvement of the community in the creation of the unit and education about its purpose would have helped shape appropriate perceptions of the purpose. Proper selection and orientation of the new manager (including a different selection process) as well as orientation of all of the unit staff would have made a difference. The multitude of interpersonal conflicts that occurred were not rooted in personal differences. The systemic problem was inadequate attention to the creation and implementation of purpose.

Structure refers to ensuring that the organization is designed to carry out the purposes and the work. "Form follows function" is a wise guideline in deciding how to structure. A common mistake in structuring is to have a familiar or preferred structure in mind and then fit the work into it. While there is rarely one way to do anything in human systems—a concept known as "equifinality" (Katz and Kahn 1966)—that does not mean that any way will do. Organization design is a popular topic now, precisely because most people who manage complex organizations are struggling with how best to organize in order to get the work done most effectively. Contemporary technology, democratization of the workplace, increasing interdependence, virtual organizations, etc., make structure very confusing. Structure refers to how the work is divided up and then, of course, how to coordinate and control those interdependent parts. It is important to remember that there is no perfect structure.

Return again to our example of the newly established EPS unit. The work as defined by the mission or purpose of the organization was to provide time-limited services to resolve crises and refer clients to other resources for further treatment. The manager could divide up the work on the basis of the function served—psychiatrists, nurses, psychologists, social workers, and administrative assistants. Or staff could be grouped around the service provided by forming an interdisciplinary mix of each of the functional groups. Limited specialist resources such as diagnosis and consultation could be retained as a separate group available as needed by service-providing groups. Coordination and control could be centralized by having direct reporting to the manager or decentralized to service-providing groups who operate within unit guidelines established by the manager. Each organization will determine what is best for its circumstance, taking into account factors like mission or purpose, patient load, nature of crises presented (related in part to the nature of the catchment area), number and qualifications of resources available to the unit, etc. The point here is that preconceived notions of what a structure should look like are often not useful. The structure must fit the work and the situation.

Another example is the case of an ambulatory care program in a state mental hospital that is mandated to address the homeless population. A traditional functional and hierarchical structure may have to give way to a decentralized community-based organization organized around multidisciplinary teams. Matrix relationships provide professional supervision and support, while a central management team coordinates the overall program.

Each structure has advantages and disadvantages. In thinking through and choosing a structure, anticipate the disadvantages and do whatever is possible to address them. For example, matrix structures (where people have more than one boss and/or have responsibility but not authority) are especially useful in organizations with complex technology and project-type work (hospitals) but are sure to generate conflict. The enlightened manager will know that the conflict in this case is largely a product of the structure and will support the structure with things like periodic coordinating meetings, training in negotiation skills, and reward systems that reinforce collaboration.

Structure rarely stays in place very long in today's organizations. As the work and direction of the organization change, it is often sensible to adjust or even rethink the structure in order to ensure that it helps (not hinders) carrying out the work. After the structure has been selected from the several possible alternatives (to force thinking and debate), it is up to the manager to make it work. Most often, that means that he or she must be the major force for keeping the organization integrated. While it is a hackneyed concept, "management by walking around" (Peters and Waterman 1982) is of enormous value in learning about problems before they become dilemmas and for keeping the interdependent people and groups in contact with one another. **No structure will be so elegant as to preclude the constant need for making it work.**

The **Relationships** box refers to the way individuals and work units interact. Where people need to work together, they must do it well. It is less important if the individuals or the work units are not interdependent—that is, do not have to cooperate in order for either of them to do their work effectively. The manager should first assess the amount of interdependency involved when there are relationship problems. That will determine the seriousness and need or priority for intervention. Some technologies (e.g., administration and medicine) will be in constant tension. At least some of that tension is desirable in order to ensure that each does its job and stays focused on its task. This kind of tension is not likely to be eliminated, nor should it be. **The way conflict is managed is as important as the presence of conflict itself.** For reasons assumed to be well understood by the audience of this book, conflict is loaded with psychodynamics, and they are heightened by authority relations. The way conflict is managed—much more than the presence of conflict—is a key ingredient in the formation and existence of organization culture. Culture is a powerful force and one that can be relied upon to override individual judgment. The culture provides—and limits—many individual choices about how to behave in the organization.

A useful checklist in managing conflict in the organization is as follows:

1. **understand that conflict exists and must be managed between individuals, groups, and kinds of work;**
2. **some conflict should exist and not be suppressed if it is important for each party to stay clear about its particular purpose;**
3. **it is most important to attend to conflict where the people or groups must cooperate in order for either of them to do their work well;**

4. **some conflict may be caused by unclear direction setting or by the structure;**
5. **the part that is not dealt with by preceding advice on managing those variables needs to be addressed with individuals and groups involved;**
6. **the way all conflict between key individuals and groups is managed sets the tone for managing differences and creating the culture for everyone else in the entire organization;**
7. **the manager is responsible for how conflict is managed; it is essential that the manager be objective—for example, not favor the person, function, or group that the manager used to be a part of.**

As an example of items 6 and 7, consider the case of a planning committee in a hospital. The members of the committee represent various professional specialties, and each member is interested in garnering scarce resources (e.g., beds, OR time, diagnostic equipment) for his or her part of the system. The chairperson does not want to confront the differences expressed in the meetings and makes one-to-one deals outside the meetings. As a result the larger system goes unattended, since the work of the group becomes individual maneuvering by members with the chairperson. That person's power is exaggerated, and power politics becomes the norm, which soon becomes the culture of the organization. Members of the committee do not take responsibility for the larger system and do not try to balance it. Instead, they try to maximize their part of it.

No one is exempt from difficulties in addressing conflict situations. The manager plays a key role in setting the tone and modeling effective conflict management behavior. Peter Block (1981) advocates "moving toward the tension," since most people avoid it. As a person, you too may wish to avoid conflict in the organization. As a manager, you have a responsibility to move toward it and manage it. Conflict can be avoided, suppressed, and smoothed over or else confronted and worked through to agreed-upon actions. The first step in intervening in conflict situations is to work with the individuals or groups involved and reach an agreed-upon definition of the problem. It is possible that the conflict involves different views of purpose or goals or differences about the way work is divided up or coordinated (structure). In these cases the preceding discussion about these issues can be useful. Do not hesitate to seek training in conflict management. Several references that are useful in learning about managing conflict are:

Managing Conflict: Interpersonal Dialogue and Third Party Roles, by Richard Walton (Reading, MA: Addison-Wesley, 1987)

Getting to Yes: Negotiating Agreement without Giving In, by Roger

Fisher, William Ury, and Bruce Patton (New York: Penguin Books, 1991)

(See references for full citation.)

Your human resources officer can also provide you with information on readings, workshops, and/or consultation. It is essential to keep the larger system perspective in mind when dealing with conflict situations. That is, seek the outcome that will best serve the larger unit or organization's purpose and goals.

The **Rewards** box is usefully divided into two parts—reward and reinforcement. Reward refers to the longer-term performance period, say twelve months, at the end of which one's performance is evaluated and rewarded by merit pay, bonus, or longer-term incentive. Salary, benefits, and reward, as defined here, most likely will encourage high performance if they are seen as symbols of high-quality work valued by the organization. Rewards frequently get diluted in motivational value over time, however, and become expected or do not truly discriminate among different performance levels. It is well to remember that a satisfied need is not a motivator.

Reinforcement refers to the day-to-day shaping of behavior by recognizing and providing psychological as well as tangible encouragement of incremental behavior. Certainly, appreciation, when earned, is appropriate as well as being a useful reinforcement. The more specific the recognition, the more valuable it is as a motivator. "Good job, Bill" is not as useful as "Bill, the plan you created for that project, the agendas, and the conduct of the three monitoring meetings as well as the measurements you devised really helped to make that project a success." This is an area in which knowing the individual is an asset. Some people are fueled by recognition from authority figures; some get more from increased responsibility; some like being able to learn new skills. Use what works best for the individual. Most of all, reward what the organization says it rewards; for example, getting work done, demonstrating the desired organization values, and taking responsibility. Few managers can control the reward system. They administer parts of established programs. **All managers, however, have complete control of the reinforcement system or the day-to-day shaping of behavior.**

Opportunities for reinforcement and reward are often missed. For example, attending a training program (especially if it is in a nice place) can be a reward initiated by the boss rather than a request granted by the boss to an employee pleading a case to attend. Tying rewards to development is essential. For example, development and use of skills in communication, collaboration, and group decision making is not likely if rewards and reinforcement are only on the basis of individual professional and technical competence.

Rewarding and reinforcing how the work is done as well as what is done is important. For example, rewarding someone who accomplishes work at the expense of others or by monopolizing scarce resources does not build an effective organization or group culture.

Rewards is another area in which you will need counsel and interaction with the Human Resources function. It is well to remember that the work itself should be a reward by being a source of psychic income. This means that jobs should inherently contain opportunities for things like achievement, feedback, responsibility, and recognition (Herzberg et al. 1959; Hackman and Oldham 1980).

Helpful Mechanisms includes traditional management systems like planning, budgeting, control, and measurements. These systems have a great deal to do with organization behavior. For example, performance management (the individual objective-setting process part) must be integrated with organization planning and budgeting to ensure that individuals will have the prerequisite context of organization and unit goals from the planning process in order to set their objectives. Resources must be available from the budgeting process to carry out the objectives. Otherwise, individual work, no matter how diligently pursued, will not contribute to larger organization efforts.

Helpful mechanisms also include formal things like policies, procedures, and meetings as well as informal things like bulletin boards, lunch gatherings, and even social events. Informal mechanisms can be created rather than leaving them to chance. One organization intentionally put comfortable benches near water fountains and other gathering places as a way of encouraging people to talk. Some managers feared it would encourage idling, but that did not happen. Whether formal or informal, the question to ask continually about any mechanism is "Is it helpful?" For example, a budgeting or performance management system that is not helpful needs attention. Helpful mechanisms and leadership are important integrators of organization behavior.

The **Leadership** box is a critical one because the way the leader behaves is of such consequence to the behavior of others in the organization. Here the words *manager* and *leader* are used interchangeably even though much has been said about the differences in recent years. Rather than examining the traits or styles of leaders, the emphasis here is on the work of the leader. While much has been written about the work of leaders, a classic article by Selznick (1957) identifies **four tasks that must be performed by a leader in order to make the system as a whole operate effectively.** They are:

1. **Defining purpose** (and direction-setting, as discussed previously)
2. **Ensuring that programs exist for purposes** (turn the aims into action)
3. **Defending institutional integrity** (ensure that the organization meets external needs and stays healthy)
4. **Ordering internal conflict** (that critical role of conflict management).

In addition, leaders must balance the other boxes. An effective work system optimizes all of the parts instead of maximizing any of them. In a hospital physicians want to maximize medical delivery; administrators want to maximize financial health; medical technologists want to maximize the technical systems. The leader balances the competing desires for getting the most for their part with a view toward the effectiveness of the larger system. This may be done by allocating resources in a seemingly unfair way. For example, salary increases for people who do a particular kind of work may be necessary in order to compete in a tight labor market, or membership in some decision-making process may need to be altered to insert a necessary point of view. As always, **leadership carries with it the role of modeling and setting the tone in all aspects of organization work and life.**

Change in any part (or box) affects some or all of the other parts. For example, change in mission and key goals may dictate a review of structure to ensure that the current function is not being carried out by a form designed for a different function. Change in structure may necessitate work on the rewards system to ensure that the behaviors desired in the structure are appropriately encouraged by rewards and reinforcements. Change in leadership—or the kind of leadership—can affect everything. This is illustrated by the fact that most organization change efforts that terminate prematurely or do not become institutionalized are related to changes in leadership where the new leader is not supportive of the change or operates inappropriately in it.

Diagnosing the Organization

One of the many uses of an organization model is that it provides a framework for diagnosis. You may wish to conduct a diagnosis because you sense something is systematically dysfunctional or because you simply want to monitor the general health of the system. In either case you can use this organization model to answer your questions.

The variables or component parts of the model enable you to concentrate your focus, after which you can examine the relationship between the parts. Follow the sequence in which the variables are presented here—that is, start with purpose/direction setting, followed by structure, etc. If you are examining the larger system or a major component such as a significant department or function, think of the questions needing to be asked in each variable. For example, if you are diagnosing the Purposes or Direction Setting box of the hospital (the larger system) you would want to find out things like:

1. **What purpose(s) do we serve? (mission)**
2. **Who are our clients/customers?**
3. **How well are we accomplishing our mission?**
4. **What are our priority goals for the operating year?**
5. **Are subunit goals aimed at accomplishing the hospital goals?**
6. **Are those goals understood and agreed upon by key subunit managers?**
7. **Do individuals in those units have objectives aimed at accomplishing unit goals?**

Taking each of the variables in sequence, you can involve key managers in whatever level of the system is being diagnosed in deciding what to inquire about, from whom, and how (survey, interview, focus groups, etc.). If you are a group manager, working at a lower level of the system, you would approach the task the same way but ask questions appropriate to your level of the system. You would likely start with the purpose of the group and its goals, then ask how your group is supporting the accomplishment of the larger system mission and goals, etc.

Organization diagnosis is an extremely useful concept for managers, and most will need to learn more about the subject or use an external or internal organization development consultant to do anything other than an overview diagnosis. In addition to Weisbord, a recommended reading in this area is *Diagnosis for Organizational Change: Methods and Models,* by Ann Howard and Associates (1994).

Organizations are open systems and continually redefine themselves as they interact with their environment. An organization is embedded in a society and community, an industry, and an economy. A subunit of an organization is embedded in a larger organization, and a work group is embedded in a department that is embedded in a larger organization. Because of these environments, it is usually wise to expand a problem and ask, "What is that problem connected to?" in order to truly define an organizational problem. For example, a manager may define performance appraisal as a problem. Expanding the problem, we see that appraisal is connected to objective setting, which is related to the planning process.

After analysis it may be that appraisal is not so much the problem as is the problem of setting useful individual objectives when the planning process does not make unit goals and budgets available at the time when individual objectives are negotiated.

While managing organization behavior (primarily by managing the contextual variables that lead to a lot of the individual behavior) is complex, we have been using the existing organization as a reference. What about the issues involved in managing organization behavior when the organization is changing?

Managing Organization Change

Because change is now the constant state for organizations, it has received a lot of study. Change is now divided into categories, which are:

1. **First-Order Change**—also known as incremental change. This refers to the alteration of organization characteristics by some degrees. Examples are adding a new incentive program to the compensation system, rearranging reporting relationships in a new configuration of an existing structure, or changing work unit goals to fit new conditions.
2. **Second-Order Change**—also known as fundamental change or transformational change. This refers to a shift in basic understanding of the organization. Examples are changing the mission, changing compensation philosophy (e.g., from salary to incentive), or creating a new structure (e.g., from functionally based to matrix or changing the organization's strategic goals).

Some would say that transformational change is also defined by movement into the unknown, which makes it more difficult (Reddy 1994). For our purposes we will use *incremental* and *fundamental* for the two basic kinds of change. While strategies for managing organization behavior differ with the two kinds of change, the approach taken here is that the principles are common (e.g., the use of participation), and fundamental change is becoming so prevalent that it is probably the more useful overall template to use.

Kurt Lewin (1958) developed a model for change that is useful at any level of the system—individual, group, or organization. Simply stated, the model is: Unfreeze—Change—Refreeze. Let us examine that three-phase model more closely because its simplicity belies its profundity.

Unfreezing refers to readiness for change. An organization will not be able to change unless it has a readiness or motivation arising from things like poor performance, poor morale, or a need to acquire (or be acquired by) another organization in order to remain viable. Readiness for change often means feeling enough pain in order to be willing to accept the difficult task of major change. Sometimes the awareness of a more desirable future state can create a readiness. Unfreezing is where letting go of existing beliefs occurs. We have already discussed the value of creating a clear purpose and direction in order to manage organization behavior. This is equally true in managing change. People will not let go of what they have until they can see what to hold on to, which is the basis of vision-driven change.

Unfreezing often means disconfirming existing views or realities. For example, if people believe they are providing appropriate services, they will resist changing those services. They must have information or experience that disconfirms their belief that they are providing appropriate services. The best way to do this is to involve them in some sort of data collection to surface the issue. They could be asked to do a customer service or quality research effort in which they would be involved in deciding what information to collect, from whom, and how. Matching that information against the organization's mission or purpose and asking, "Are we accomplishing our purpose or stated reason for being?" can lead to questioning current programs and services, which can disconfirm the belief that existing ones are appropriate. It is important not to have an outsider design the data collection effort, conduct it, and report back, since that person will simply become a messenger to be shot and reinforce the belief of group or organization members that "we're OK." Appropriate consulting help would be used to work collaboratively with the members to help them design, collect, and interpret the data.

Unfreezing can also be accomplished when people experience guilt or anxiety by understanding that a gap exists between the present state and the desired state. In any event unfreezing will not occur if people believe they are at risk, for example, viewing decisions made in the past as wrong. Any disconfirming activity to create readiness or motivation must protect members' self-esteem or the esteem of others.

Change, or movement, is the intervention phase that moves the organization from its previous state to the desired one. This includes planning what needs to be done and how to implement the change. Effective change is planned change. This is the period of transition from what was to what will be. Again, a well-defined vision of the future state is essential here. The tasks needing to be accomplished for the change to occur must be defined, management mechanisms (e.g., task forces, coordinating bodies) must be created to accomplish the tasks, strategies must be developed to obtain commitment from key players, communications strategies and mechanisms must be created and resources, experts, and consultants to assist in the transition must be put in place. This is what is meant by managing the transition (Beckhard and Pritchard 1992), or the change part of Lewin's theory.

If appropriate staff have been involved in creating the readiness for change, and are themselves motivated to consider change, they are well positioned to use the data collected and conclusions drawn from it to ask, "What might we do to close the gap or achieve the desired state?" Joint action planning not only creates possible action steps but engages key members in accepting and working toward the change. It is common to see temporary groups created within the organization to think through and recommend action steps. Doing this enables people to take responsibility and identify with the new state. Compare this to a consulting firm that comes into the organization at the request of top management (and is often a mystery or threat to everyone else) and tells the organization what its problems are and what to do about them. Many such reports that cost enormous amounts of money sit unused on managers' bookshelves.

Refreezing means doing what is necessary to stabilize the new state and behavior. Many writers about organization change recommend establishing guardians of the new culture—carefully selected leaders who model the new culture and are charged with keeping others aware of it. The rewards system is important in institutionalizing change because it can reinforce the desired behaviors.

Refreezing also means institutionalizing the new state or building it into the infrastructure of the group or organization. This is where the organization model is useful. Taking each of the six boxes one can ask what can be done to encourage the change. One thing that is clear throughout Lewin's model is the value of data in making change, from unfreezing to refreezing. Lewin referred to the role and importance of data-based change as Action Research, where no data was collected unless there was a commitment to act on it and no action was taken without data. In the refreezing step it is essential to build in ongoing data collection to monitor the effects of the changes made. This also keeps the organization more able to adapt to the inevitability of ongoing change. This is the essence of the popular concept of the "learning organization" (Senge 1990).

Some argue that the environment is so turbulent today that there is no refreezing phase. Yet the need for psychological closure with humans is such that, even if there is not refreezing, it is important to mark the attainment of a "changing new state." The three stages of Lewin's change theory are not discrete steps and probably better described as phases where overlap occurs. Few behavioral models involving sequential or predictable movement, such as stages of group development, are able to be divided into discrete steps. **Organization change is always messy, never neat, and the effective change agent is one who can work with messiness.**

Refer again to our example of the new EPS unit. It is clear that not much attention was paid to unfreezing or ensuring the readiness for change. Gatekeepers, in Lewin's terms, would be people like the new unit director, the chief of psychiatry at the hospital, key clinical and administrative people there, and some community leaders. Useful data to collect would include existing perceptions of services provided, services needed but not provided, the purposes of the proposed unit, its relationship to the hospital, staff and competencies required. The gatekeepers would be in charge of the data to collect and the analysis of the data. Prior to collecting data, there must be clarity about how decisions regarding its use would be made (e.g., by consensus, by authority, or by selected individuals) and by whom (e.g., managers only or managers and community leadership).

The change phase would be where the purposes or mission of the new EPS unit would be developed. The desired state of the new unit when the unit is up and running would be described. A transition plan that describes how the gap between the existing state and the desired state would be developed. Human resources systems such as performance management and compensation would be reviewed to ensure that they support the desired state. A communication plan—very important—would be developed to ensure that people in the hospital, the new unit, and the community would be continuously aware of what was taking place. Forums for information exchange and dialogue would be created. The structure of the unit would be established. All of these activities would likely be done by temporary groups that included relevant people in the hospital (including Human Resources and Psychiatry), the new unit, and the community. The managers in the organization who will implement the change will need support as the change is implemented. All of this would be overseen by a coordinating group of managers senior enough to support the work of others by removing roadblocks and obtaining resources.

Refreezing (to the extent that this occurs today) would be accomplished by establishing performance measurements for the new organization, monitoring, and acting on them. The supporting systems mentioned previously, such as individual performance management and compensation, would be continually monitored and aligned to support the desired state and high organizational performance. Ongoing diagnosis of the organization using the variables described earlier can be a form of monitoring. This ongoing monitoring becomes a way of developing a learning organization. In short, the culture of the new organization is built so the change is not left to the determined effort of individuals.

Resistance to change is a major issue in the planning and implementation of organization change. The tendency is to speed toward change once it has been decided upon. A useful formula (Beckhard and Harris 1987) for anticipating resistance to change is:

$C = (A + B + D) > X$, where

C = Change
A = Level of dissatisfaction with the status quo
B = Desirability of the proposed change or end state
D = Practicality of the change (minimal risk and disruption)
X = Cost of changing.

The authors say that

> factors A, B and D must outweigh the perceived costs (X) for change to occur. If any person or group whose commitment is needed is not sufficiently dissatisfied with the present state of affairs (A), eager to achieve the proposed end state (B) and convinced about the feasibility of the change (D), then the cost (X) of changing is too high, and that person or group will resist the change. (Beckhard and Pritchard 1992)

It is critically important to diagnose the readiness for change and do whatever is necessary, collect whatever data is needed, educate and communicate about the present state of the organization, and ensure that all of the key people who will be involved in the change truly understand the need for it. They must agree that it is worth the cost of the change. Many a change effort has failed at this point. Even though the change was, on the surface, implemented quickly, no change in fact occurred even though people went through the motions.

Four of the most common reasons, given by Kotter and Schlesinger (1979), **that people resist change are:**

1. **A desire not to lose something of value**
2. **A misunderstanding of the change and its implementation**
3. **A belief that the change does not make sense for the organization**
4. **A low tolerance for change**

People understandably focus on their own interests. They may, for example, perceive a potential loss in status or power as a result of the change. They may fear they will not be able to do what is required of them in the new state or may believe that support of the change would be an admission that some of their previous decisions or beliefs were in error. There are many ways in which individuals can perceive the change as a threat.

Most managers vastly underestimate both the many ways in which resistance can be manifest as well as their ability to constructively address the resistance. Kotter and Schlesinger provide **tips on dealing with the four kinds of resistance** they identified. Some of their recommendations are:

1. **Education and Communication**
2. **Participation and Involvement**
3. **Facilitation and Support**

As stated in the preceding example, educating and communicating with people about the need for the change is essential. This can take the form of seminars, one-to-one discussions, informal talks (e.g., at lunch), written documents, videotapes, teleconferences, and Internet communications. **Personal contact with authority figures, especially the boss, is the best form of education.** This is why key managers must be committed to the change before reaching out to others. One cannot fake commitment to change—that is all too detectable. **Be assured that the amount of education and communication needed is always, always, underestimated.** The guidelines here are: **(1) Communicate, (2) Communicate,** and **(3) Communicate. Key managers must be personally involved, especially when there are difficult issues involved.**

As described in the unfreezing phase discussions, participation and involvement of potential resisters early on will pay large dividends. Identify resisters who are key to the change before proceeding, involve them in the design and implementation of the effort. Also, listen and take advice from those who do the work. They will always know something that the change planners do not. In general, participation helps gain commitment. Some managers are resistant to any participation, and some believe everyone should participate in everything. We are talking here about appropriate participation. Remember that participation in identifying issues and planning change strategies does not necessarily mean that those same people participate in decision making. The more people who can, appropriately, be involved in decision making, the better. Coordination and control is not lost by involving people in thinking through and understanding change issues. There is seldom reason why some form of involvement is not possible.

Facilitation and support can take the form of listening and being emotionally supportive, or it can be tangible, such as providing training. Cutting some slack in the work rules when people are coping with change—for example, attendance or time off—can help. When the resistance is rooted in fear of performing poorly in the new state, skill training and education costs are good investments. **When planning for change, anticipate things like time required for communication and education, time required for listening, and money required for training, education, and counseling.**

Since many activities will be going on simultaneously, **it is advisable to create a coordinating committee** like the one in the example to ensure that the activities are integrated and result in the desired total system change. While it might be seen in the traditional sense as a steering committee, it has more complex responsibilities, which include:

1. **Viewing the change from the system (vs-part) level**
2. **Ensuring that system-wide and system-level communication occurs**
3. **Balancing the change activities for the benefit of the system (e.g., allocating resources appropriately)**
4. **Setting the tone and creating the culture for the change.**

It is important that this group keep in mind that the parts of the system are related. Change in any part affects the other parts. Leaving the change interventions to the individual parts of the organization can result in duplicate efforts, canceling out of efforts, competition, and larger system failure. One might compare this group to the family practice physician who monitors and integrates the work of specialists.

Summary

Managing organization behavior can often mean taking your eye off the person who is acting out the organization dynamics and looking instead at the organization itself. This means that managers need to understand what an organization is, its component parts, how they interact, and how the context of the organization can affect individual behavior. Before intervening with individuals, examine the group and organizational context, for example, to ensure that the person understands and agrees with the purposes and goals. The way conflict is managed is a major factor in creating the culture of an organization. Conflict management is, therefore, a major responsibility of managers.

Since change can be assumed to be a constant in today's organizations, managing change is essential for managing organization behavior. **Having a concept for change and its dynamics is essential for good managing.** Often, organizational change is implemented before establishing a readiness for change. Data are required. Involving key people in collecting and interpreting data is essential throughout the change process, from creating readiness to planning of change to implementation and monitoring. Resistance to change is part of change. Anticipating and dealing with resistance is part of planning for change. It cannot be overemphasized that appropriate use of consultants who work in organization change will pay dividends. While communication, education, participation, and training are necessary, individual training is never a change strategy; it supports change strategy. To change an organization, one must change the context in which individuals live and work.

There are many theories of organization change. Although Lewin was aware of and accounted for unconscious behavior, this chapter did not refer much to psychodynamic theories such as those of Kernberg (1978), Kaplan (1974), Levinson (1972), and Hirshhorn (1989). **The particular theory or theories used are not as important as being sure you are operating from a concept and not reacting intuitively or shooting from the hip.** As stated in the opening of this chapter, managing organizational behavior is a complex task and requires a disciplined and thoughtful approach.

GLOSSARY

Change Movement from current state to future state—hopefully the desired future state

Diagnosis Data collected and analyzed to prepare people to act and to provide baseline data on the present state in order to compare it to the desired state; diagnosis is only done if one is prepared to make necessary changes

Direction setting Clarifying and articulating the aim of organization work at any level of the system, from organization purpose or mission to individual objectives

Helpful mechanisms Anything that helps coordinate the organizational system from traditional control and coordination systems such as budgeting and planning to monthly meetings or hallway bulletin boards

Leadership Work done by anyone who has the role or opportunity to define direction and align individual and group efforts to achieve it

Organization An open system of related parts that continually redefines itself as it interacts with its environment

Refreezing Making the future state the norm or "the way things are done here"

Reinforcement Benefit accrued to a person at any time (e.g., praise for a task well done or an on-the-spot cash award)

Relationships The way in which individuals and work units interact, especially in regard to how conflict is managed

Resistance to change The natural state of not wanting to let go of what is currently valued or understood—even if it is only "the devil I know!"—will exist unless attention to the unfreezing and change processes are done well

Rewards Benefit accrued to a person at the end of a defined period of time (e.g., bonus at end of year)

Structure The division of labor and the authority and coordination necessary to integrate it in order to achieve the purpose of the organization

Unfreezing Getting people ready for change

Work group People collaborating on a task

REFERENCES

Beckhard, R., and R. T. Harris. 1987. *Managing Complex Change,* 2d ed. Reading, MA: Addison-Wesley.

Beckhard, R., and W. Pritchard. 1992. *Changing the Essence: The Art of Creating and Leading Fundamental Change in Organizations.* San Francisco: Jossey-Bass.

Block, P. 1981. Flawless Consulting. Austin, TX: Learning Concepts.

Burke, W.W. 1992. *Organization Development: A Process of Learning and Changing.* Reading, MA: Addison-Wesley.

Fisher, R., W. Ury, and B. Patton. 1991. *Getting to Yes: Negotiating Agreement without Giving In,* 2d ed. New York: Penguin Books.

Gump, L. R. 1983. Behaviorism and human resource development: Paradox and prospects. MS. Annapolis, MD: BDR Learning Products.

Hackman, J. R., and G. R. Oldham. 1980. *Work Redesign.* Reading, MA: Addison-Wesley.

Herzberg, F., B. Mausner, and B. B. Snyderman. 1959. *The Motivation to Work.* New York: Wiley.

Hirshhorn, L. 1988. *The Workplace Within: Psychodynamics of Organization Life.* Cambridge, MA: MIT Press.

Howard, Ann, and Associates. 1994. *Diagnosis for Organizational Change: Methods and Models.* New York: Guilford Press.

Kaplan, S. R. 1974. Characteristic phases of development in organizations. In D. Millman and G. Goldman, eds., *Group Process Today, Evaluation and Perspectives.* Springfield, IL: Thomas.

Katz, D., and R. L. Kahn. 1966. *The Social Psychology of Organizations.* New York: John Wiley and Sons.

Kernberg, O. 1978. Leadership and organizational functioning: Organization regression. *International Journal of Group Psychotherapy* 29:3–25.

Kotter, J. P., and L. A. Schlesinger. 1979. Choosing strategies for change. *Harvard Business Review* (March–April).

Levinson, H. 1972. *Organizational Diagnosis.* Cambridge, MA: Harvard University Press.

Lewin, K. 1958. Group decisions and social change. *Readings in Social Psychology.* New York: Holt, Rinehart and Winston.

Morrow, A. F. 1969. *The Practical Theorist.* Annapolis, MD: BDR Learning Products.

Peters, T. J., and R. H. Waterman. 1982. *In Search of Excellence.* New York: Harper and Row.

Reddy, B. W. 1994. *Intervention Skills: Process Consultation for Small Groups and Trainers.* San Diego: Pfeiffer and Co.

Selznick, P. 1957. *Leadership in Administration.* New York: Harper and Row.

Senge, P. 1990. *The Fifth Discipline.* New York: Doubleday.

Walton, R. E. 1987. *Managing Conflict: Interpersonal Dialogue and Third Party Roles,* 2d ed. Reading, MA: Addison-Wesley.

Weisbord, M. R. 1978. *Organizational Diagnosis: A Workbook of Theory and Practice.* Reading, MA: Addison-Wesley.

CHAPTER 9

Human Resources in Mental Health Care Organizations

William F. Martin, Psy.D., M.P.H., M.A.

The mental health industry gradually and quietly transformed from a cottage industry of independent solo practices into a conglomerate of solo practices affiliated with large mental health care organizations and independent group practices. Recently, the mental health industry has become dominated by a few organizational players. Grazier (1998) discovered that the four largest mental health care organizations control about 60 percent of the managed behavioral health care market. Moreover, more than half (60 percent) of the U.S. population is enrolled in a managed behavioral health care plan (Grazier 1998). These huge shifts in the mental health industry place a tremendous amount of pressure on mental health care organizations, their leaders and managers, as well as the practitioners who provide services to the millions of patients who utilize mental health services.

Mental health care organizations are faced with numerous challenges as health care continues to change with respect to delivery, financing, regulations, quality, and technology. The rate and amount of change that will confront mental health care administrators will steadily increase as the twenty-first century unfolds. Those mental health administrators that realize the source of adaptation, care, innovation, satisfaction, and service will be the administrators who will lead their practices and mental health care organizations to a viable place in the increasingly competitive marketplace.

What is the source of adaptation, care, innovation, satisfaction, and service? Accountants and financial experts will tell you that the source is cost accounting, capital budgeting, sophistical reimbursement schemes, and creative financing deals. Attorneys will suggest that the source is savvy contracting, negotiating, mediating, settling, and even, litigation. Operational aficionados will demonstrate with sound evidence that the source is streamlined operations designed to maximize efficiency and effectiveness.

Health care providers will share with you that high quality care is the source along with excellent customer service. Marketing and sales professionals will suggest that the source is vision-oriented marketing plans with aggressive sales force tactics that identify niches to exploit.

The source is all of these. A deeper level of analysis, however, is required. The common theme that runs through all of the functions outlined here is the individual and collective talent, dedication, and energy of the human resources that work in mental health care organizations. Everything that happens in any mental health care organization happens because of the individuals that work in the organization and the individuals that they serve as patients. **In short, the source of competitive advantage is people.**

People as a Source of Competitive Advantage

Mental health care organizations are labor-intensive and knowledge-producing organizations. Intellectual capital is the commodity that distinguishes a high-performing organization from a low-performing organization. Most mental health care organizations exist in a similar environment with respect to laws, regulations, and financing options. Moreover, most mental health care organizations employ similar diagnostic, treatment, and operational strategies. The key difference, however, is the unique abilities, perspectives, and experience of the staff of any given mental health care organization. **People are the source of competitive advantage.**

Seasoned administrators know the power of referral sources. Some clinicians can make or break a mental health care organization on the basis of their reputation, referral network, and perceived credibility. As such, it is not uncommon for mental health care organizations to steal high-producing clinicians from a competing organization. Clinicians in mental health care organizations function in two roles: sales force and provider of services sold.

Strategic Human Resources Management

Mental health administrators are typically concerned with positioning their organizations in the marketplace such that two goals are achieved: survival and prosperity. As such, the human resources role should be strategic (Rosenbluth and Peters 1998). The competitive positioning of mental health care organizations depends upon a rigorous analysis of both the external environment and the internal operations of the organization. A commonly employed tool is a SWOT analysis (internal strengths and weaknesses; external opportunities and threats). The strategic manage-

External Opportunities	**External Threats**
• What opportunities exist in the labor market to attract and retain the most competent and caring professionals?	• What threats exist outside the walls of the mental health care organization that might place the organization at risk?
Internal Strengths	**Internal Weaknesses**
• What are the individual and collective competencies of the work force? • What are the processes and ideal organization design strategies to tap into the intellectual capital of the work force?	• What are the obstacles and barriers that prevent individuals and groups from fully contributing to the organization, caring for patients, and serving customers? • What are the legal and regulatory risks involved in the management of human resources?

Fig. 1. SWOT analysis of human resources dimension

ment of human resources necessitates that mental health practitioners perform a SWOT to analyze the human resources dimension of their practice or organization. Figure 1 is a template for a SWOT analysis.

A SWOT analysis enables practitioners to develop strategies for their organizations to survive and prosper. The completion of a SWOT is referred to as the strategy development phase of strategic human resources management. After the SWOT is completed, then the strategy is developed using the questions listed in table 1. Strategy provides a mental health care organization with a direction and a course. Strategies in organizations typically are formulated within the context of the vision, mission, and values of the practice and the organization. In the case of a solo practitioner the vision of the practitioner and the solo practice are probably very similar. The same may be true for large organizations if the founders are still in control.

The next and most neglected phase of strategic human resources management is the execution of the strategies. Many mental health care organizations are very adept at developing and publishing strategic plans but

TABLE 1. Strategy Development Questions Based upon SWOT Analysis

Key Strategy Development Questions
How can we exploit the external opportunities before our competitors (first-mover advantage)?
How can we minimize our external threats and/or reduce our risk exposure?
How can we maintain our internal strengths?
How can we improve our internal weaknesses?

falter on the implementation of such plans. Strategic execution only happens by fully utilizing all of the human resources available to the organization. **People make strategies happen.**

One of the best ways to execute strategies is to address the fundamental question to workers: What's in it for me? The response to this question can make the difference between a mental health care organization that is on course and one that is drifting in the rough and turbulent waters of a health care monsoon. The single most effective way to execute human resources strategies is to align the strategies with operational plans, department plans, team plans, and individual performance plans. For instance, a mental health care organization that has developed a strategy to increase outpatient market share in dementia assessments will have to make sure that the organization's operational plan includes this goal, that the appropriate departmental plans share this goal, and that competent staff will be held accountable for increasing the market share and providing the dementia assessments. Alignment is a shortcut to strategy execution and a well-guided organization. **Alignment is the rudder of the corporate ship.**

Role and Functions of Human Resources Management: A Systems Approach

Human resources in mental health care organizations plays several key roles. First, human resources is responsible for recruiting, selecting, staffing, compensating, orienting, training, disciplining, rewarding, recognizing, and terminating employees, contractors, and other workers. All of these responsibilities represent the core functions of human resources. Second, human resources is accountable for minimizing exposure to legal liabilities and other liabilities. Third, human resources is increasingly becoming needed to align the vision, mission, values, strategies, and operations with the people functions of the organization.

The systems approach to human resources is grounded in concepts that are similar to family systems theory and Gestalt theory. Specifically, the whole of human resources is greater than the sum of the individual functions constituting human resources. As such, it is critical that administrators think systematically when dealing with any single human resources related issue because a change in compensation can inadvertently result in a grievance or even a lawsuit. One of the key questions to ask when thinking systematically: **What are the potential intended and unintended consequences of my decisions and/or actions?** A focus on the unintended consequences brings to light the interrelatedness of diverse factors that make up the human resources function of a wide range of mental health care organizations from solo practices to multidisciplinary group practices spanning several states.

Functions

All human resources departments or processes have the core functions listed in table 2.

The size of the mental health care organization determines if the functions are handled along with the other duties of the solo practitioner or dealt with by a single human resources department or in larger organizations by a department dedicated to human resources management.

Regardless of the size of the human resources department, it is critical that the organization of the human resources functions be designed in a

TABLE 2. Core Human Resources Functions

Functions	Overall Responsibility
Staffing	Acquire talent
Development: orientation, training, and organizational development	Socialize new employees to job and organization and invest in the current and future knowledge and skills required to reach full potential and fully contribute
Performance	Provide continuous feedback aimed at promoting excellence
Rewards and recognition	Meet the basic and higher order needs of employees
Retrenchment	Ethically respond to marketplace challenges by fully utilizing workforce and redesigning organizational structure and processes
Disciplinary	Establish development-focused systems that are legally defensible to obtain desired performance behaviors
Legal/regulatory	Communicate, educate, and comply with all laws and regulations governing organizations, employees, and unions
Labor relations	Protect the safety, welfare, and psychological well-being of all employees

way that is seamless and addresses the holistic concerns of individual employees and workers. Human resources should serve as a model of an organizational architecture that erases the silo mentality of most mental health organizations.

The silo mentality of mental health care organizations occurs when different individuals and/or departments are responsible for carrying out a prescribed set of duties and responsibilities that is necessary but not sufficient. The dilemma occurs when an assigned task or responsibility is shared by two or more practitioners and/or departments and there is some confusion about who will be held accountable and who is responsible. It is not uncommon for a game of blaming to emerge and even splitting at this point. As such, ideally designed mental health care organizations should balance division of labor with managing the white spaces between the organizational boxes.

The various functions will be presented individually for purposes of clarity. It must be noted, however, that from a systems perspective all of the functions are interrelated in a complex web of interdependencies.

Staffing Function: Forecasting, Recruitment, Selection, and Placement

The acquisition of talent is the first step in the management of intellectual capital. Mental health administrators shall become comfortable maintaining a dual focus on the here and now and the future. Futurists use several tools to forecast trends. These tools include but are not limited to the extrapolation of current events, business cycles, and scenario building.

Forecasting

Mental health organization administrators and clinicians must ask themselves some questions to forecast the future demand for mental health services and request human resources to meet that demand. Several questions are shown in table 3. The responses to these questions provide the necessary information to develop and implement a targeted recruitment campaign.

Recruitment

There are two categories of recruitment: internal and external. Promotion from within represents internal. External recruitment is searching for outsiders. Mental health care organizations prefer one mode to another. There are advantages and disadvantages to both. Table 4 illustrates the advantages and disadvantages to both.

Internal Recruitment

Strategies include job posting, career development, mentoring, and job rotation. Job posting can occur in a billboard, letter, and as a verbal exchange in a meeting. Career development is a process in which the organization has career paths. Mentoring is a socialization process of a new employee or an existing employee.

TABLE 3. Forecasting Questions

Forecasting Question	Implementation Step
What will be the epidemiological trends in the future?	Contact local and/or state health departments as well as National Institutes for Mental Health
What will be the legal and regulatory changes impacting the demand and supply of mental health labor?	Contact state mental health professional associations and organizations, labor economists, and state labor departments
What will be the supply of mental health labor in my immediate market?	Contact local mental health organizations and training programs
How can I attract talent to my mental health organization?	Conduct a 5–10-year strategic staffing plan that is aligned with the business plan and marketing plan as well as identify what candidates find attractive

TABLE 4. Advantages and Disadvantages of Internal and External Recruitment

	Internal	External
Advantages	Greater certainty of performance and "fit" Promote "from within" model tends to increase retention Basic building block of a career development program	Outside perspective Wider talent base Portrays growth with respect to public image of organization
Disadvantages	Viewed as political rather than as performance based hires Insider perspective—perhaps myopic	Greater uncertainty of performance and fit Portrays high turnover environment

External Recruitment

The acquisition of talent has become a major challenge and opportunity for all types of employers. This challenge persists even given the fact that mental health professionals are in oversupply in most fields and certainly maldistributed geographically.

Given the challenge and competition, mental health administrators should craft a planned, systematic recruitment strategy. This strategy should emphasize both passive and active approaches. Passive approaches include promoting the image of the organization and the fact that opportunities exist. Active approaches will emphasize providing training for potential candidates, participating in job fairs, advertising, and interviewing.

Selection

The goal of recruitment is to attract the most talented candidates to the organization and then proceed with a fair, legal, and powerfully predictive process to decide the best candidate for both the position and the organization. There are numerous laws, federal and state, that regulate the process of selection. These laws will be addressed in the section on **Legal/Regulatory Function.**

Selection is prediction. Selection is not fortune telling. **Selection enables administrators to make a prediction about the future performance of a candidate given a presentation of their portfolio of training and experience.** Table 5 illustrates the most common selection methods and the advantages and disadvantages of each.

The research in selection recommends that multiple methods be employed to balance the respective advantages and disadvantages of any one selection method. Yet there exists a challenge when using more than one selection method. The challenge is how to evaluate the data. There exist two basic data evaluation tools: the compensatory decision making approach and the minimum-cutoff approach.

The compensatory approach balances the strengths and weaknesses of a given candidate. For example, a candidate for a pastoral counseling position has stellar grades and outstanding recommendations but performs well below expectations during the interview. As such, the compensatory decision-making approach will weigh the credentials and recommendations higher than the job interview to compensate. In contrast, using this same example, the minimum-cutoff approach will establish minimum competencies for all selection methods. As such, poor performance on any single selection method will be evaluated as unacceptable and will result in the candidate not being selected, regardless of performance in other areas.

Development Function: Orientation, Training, and Organizational Development

The development function in human resources has become increasingly important in shaping the direction, structure, and processes of mental health organizations. A solo practitioner well knows the importance of updating knowledge and skills as behavioral health care shifts from fee-for-service to managed behavioral health care, not to mention the actual practice of mental health services from long-term approaches to short-term, brief therapy modalities.

Development is the process by which a solo practitioner or all the members of a mental health care organization stay on the cutting edge of learning in order to provide top-notch care, superb service, and to prevent the obsolescence of skills. Kaipa, Newham, and Volckmann (1998) provide a model entitled the Enterprise Pyramid. In this model business development, organizational development, knowledge development, and self-development are all aligned in an interdependent fashion. This model suggests that orientation, training, and development be viewed as an integral and core component of the organization rather than as an appendage. An illustrative example is the interrelationship between the acquisition of knowledge and the crafting of a business development strategy. **Development is ongoing.** Development does not occur in a vacuum. Development

TABLE 5. Common Selection Methods

Selection Method	Advantages	Disadvantages
Application	Easy Low-cost	Distortion
Interview	Opportunity to sell the organization Assess "fit" with culture	Subjective Legally risky
Work sample	Best predictor of future performance Realistic job preview	Expensive Time-consuming Intimidating
Behavioral event interviewing	Based on past performance Job-related questions	Task focused Investment in training interviewers

takes place within a strategic, operational, and tactical context. Development is typically divided into the following categories: orientation, training, and organizational development.

Orientation

Changes often create a sense of disorientation and can be discomforting. New employees are undergoing a change and, therefore, can benefit from being oriented to the organization, the department, their role, their position, and even their tasks. A new worker often reports to the first day of work very excited yet confused and highly motivated, yet apprehensive and educated, yet unfamiliar with how to apply their knowledge, skills, and experience in this new setting. **Orientation is a process in which new workers become more comfortable, gain clarity around the nature of their role and responsibility, and are socialized to the norms and realities of the new organization.**

Orientation should be regarded as more than simply meeting the mandates of JCAHO and NCQA. Ganzel (1998) has identified five critical success factors to an effective orientation: (1) give employees what they need to know before they ask; (2) allow sufficient time for orientation; (3) provide an immersion experience; (4) make it universal; and (5) do it now. Health care organizations have a tradition of orienting some employees and not others. It is not uncommon for health care organizations not to orient physicians, even those that are full-time, salaried employees, based upon a notion that physicians are different and that their medical school and residency experiences have provided them with all they need to know about working effectively, efficiently, and ethically in your organization. This tradition should be challenged because one of the most important reasons for orienting workers is to socialize them to the norms of the organization and to create a shared, immersion experience that is commonly held among diverse employees.

Training

Training is the acquisition of and refining of job-related knowledge and skills. Training is typically divided into training for soft skills and training for hard skills. Soft skills training are those skills required to address relationships between members of the mental health care organization and between patients and providers. Hard skills training attempts to provide workers task-focused development, for example, coding for specific diagnoses. Training can be both formal and informal.

Formal training includes courses, seminars, and workshops. Informal training includes hallway consultations, one-on-one mentoring, and coaching. **In a recent study it was found that almost 70 percent of learning in organizations takes place informally** (Day 1998). This finding provides support for building a learning organization. Peter Senge, the author of *The Fifth Discipline,* describes a learning organization as follows: "learning organizations involves developing people who learn to see as systems thinkers see, who develop their own personal mastery, and who learn how to surface and restructure mental models, collaboratively" (1990:367).

Mental health administrators have practiced the art and science of learning organizations prior to the emergence of the term itself. Case conferences, treatment plan meetings, and hallway consultations are all examples of activities that may characterize a learning organization.

Organizational Development

Orientation and training are necessary but not sufficient. Family therapists have taught us that a well child placed back into a dysfunctional family system will have a greater likelihood of manifesting dysfunctional behaviors than a well child placed in a high-functioning family system. The same principle applies to well-oriented and well-trained workers and organizational systems.

Organizational development is the art and science of creating and sustaining a well-functioning organization as a whole. The vision, mission, values, and norms are the glue that hold the structure of the organization together. There is no magic design. Yet an organization with a solid culture with support and a clear structure approaches magic.

Organizational design is necessary but not sufficient. **It has been discovered, however, that a flexible work configuration results in decreased turnover, enhanced productivity, and reduced stress** (Rosenbluth and Peters 1998). The chapter "Managing Organization Behavior" addresses the technology of organizational development in far greater detail than this chapter.

Performance Function: Performance Management System

Performance is the heart and soul of any fully functioning mental health organization. Performance represents the constellation of attitudes, behaviors, cognitions, and perceptions that are focused on achieving a specific work-related goal or set of goals. Similarly, a well-designed therapeutic system depends upon a constellation of practitioner attitudes, behaviors, cognitions, and perceptions focused on achieving a defined clinical outcome using as few resources as necessary and ethical given the unique demands of each therapeutic encounter. Diagnosis and treatment are basically ways that practitioners perform in mental health organizations. Thus, enhanced performance results in improved outcomes, increased productivity, and greater satisfaction.

A high-performing organization has an identifiable feel and energy that distinguishes it from a marginal or sub-optimal performing organization. Imagine all of the members of a jazz ensemble sitting on a stage before a packed house but not a single note can be heard. This jazz ensemble may have tremendous potential to "rock the house." Yet this pent-up potential has to be unleashed in order for the jazz ensemble to perform. Performing boils down to providing employees, patients, customers, and vendors with memorable yet satisfying experiences. Any single performance represents the tip of the iceberg. Beneath the frigid cold waters of the performance iceberg is miles and miles of practice. Practice provides the raw materials to construct the foundation of the iceberg. Practice without feedback, however, does not result in a sturdy foundation, only an illusion of stability. As such, performance management must be integrated with the tenets of organizational learning described in the preceding section on Development. Specifically, well-functioning mental health care organizations must be feedback-rich in order to survive and thrive in the twenty-first century. Accordingly, performance boils down to constructing a feedback-rich environment at all levels of the organization, from the individual practitioner to the entire organization.

Performance has to be managed in order for specific work-related goals to be achieved consistently. This should not be foreign to experienced administrators and practitioners. For example, the treatment of agoraphobia emerges from the development of a treatment plan based upon a diagnostic evaluation. Moreover, both the agoraphobic patient and the practitioner can define the nature of an effective and efficient outcome. In this particular case the outcome would be to live, work, and play in a range of outside environments while at the same time minimizing feelings of threat, anxiety, and a host of psychophysiological symptoms. At work it is critical that employees and supervisors or members of the same team know the nature of the outcomes that they seek to achieve. Furthermore, like the agoraphobic patient who has the ability to self-monitor and self-regulate his or her behavior, each and every employee must develop the capacity and be given the freedom to self-monitor and self-regulate their performance behaviors.

A subtle, more extremely important question must be posed before searching for ways to optimize the performance of individual practitioners, teams of practitioners, departments of practitioners, and even, mental health organizations: Can those in power in mental health care organizations affect the performance of others? A similar question is often posed in therapy as well: Can a practitioner affect the clinical outcome of a patient? The answers to these two central questions cannot be fully addressed in this chapter. Yet this chapter assumes that the behavior and performance of one person cannot only be influenced but even controlled by another person. **It is critical, however, that practitioners in management and leadership roles do not abuse this power but use this power to more fully develop the talents and contributions of those around them.** Also, it is essential that practitioner-managers and practitioner-leaders acknowledge the ability of all employees to control and govern themselves in pursuit of goals larger than any one individual. By acknowledging this fact, room is created for practitioner-managers and leaders to create and sustain an environment in which each employee becomes his or her own manager and leader. This is similar to the role of the practitioner who utilizes self-control as a therapeutic regimen that is based on the premise that the client's final step in treatment is "to become his or her own counselor" (Richards 1985:568).

Beyond the Annual Performance Appraisal

In many organizations the annual performance appraisal is the alpha and omega of performance management. **This is absurd.** It is just as absurd as the final report card representing the totality of feedback given to students throughout the entire school year. Yet in many organizations, the only informal and formal feedback provided to workers occurs once a year. The experience is typically dreaded by both individuals giving and receiving feedback. In addition, if the individual receiving feedback has a reputation for behaving in a defensive manner or even a threatening fashion, then the typical response of the person responsible for completing the annual performance appraisal is to procrastinate, to delay, and even to provide false feedback that highlights the positive and casts a shadow on the negative. The structure of the annual performance appraisal process promotes feelings commonly associated with confrontation and interpersonal conflict. The annual performance appraisal process has merits and drawbacks. Table 6 illustrates the merits and drawbacks of the annual performance appraisal process.

In summary, the annual performance appraisal process is necessary but not sufficient. The annual performance appraisal process should be incorporated into a total Performance Management System (PMS).

Performance Management System: Background and Description

Background

PMS manages performance in a strikingly different way than the old annual performance appraisal model. The basic differences are as follows:

PMS defines behavioral performance expectations at the beginning of the process.
PMS samples job-related behaviors throughout the entire process and feedback information continually.
PMS aligns performance functions with other functions, like compensation, development, and reward and recognition.
PMS focuses solely on performance not compensation.
PMS teaches employees to self-monitor, self-regulate, self-control, and self-reward their own performance behaviors.

These are the essential differences between PMS and the traditional performance appraisal approach. Under PMS the individual employee plays a more active role. In contrast, under the traditional annual performance

TABLE 6. Merits and Drawbacks of Annual Performance Appraisal Process

Domains	Merits	Drawbacks
Legal	Establishes legal documentation	Viewed as a legal instrument to protect organization only
Regulatory (JCAHO)	Meets JCAHO requirements	Perceived as a way to "pass" inspection only
Goal expectation setting	Clarifies goals and expectations	Communicates goals and expectations prior to performance and only at a single point in time
Performance monitoring	Monitors performance over a period of one year	Monitors performance in time increments that are too large
Feedback	Provides feedback over a period of one year	Provides feedback that is subject to rater bias

appraisal model the manager plays a more active role than the employee, who typically is the recipient of information to be refuted, defended, or challenged.

PMS is theoretically grounded in the work of Kreitner and Luthans (1984), who use Social Learning Theory as a way of describing the management of performance. Their model asserts that employees develop mental images of successful performance and then make a self-evaluation determination of their ability to perform the desired behavior (self-efficacy). An illustrative case would be an experienced psychoanalytic practitioner who has witnessed the growth of managed care in his practice. As a result, this practitioner is faced with the question and performance challenge of modifying his diagnostic and treatment behaviors to fit with the insurance coverage requirements of his patients. If this psychoanalytic practitioner decides that practicing short-term therapy is possible, then the practitioner has demonstrated self-efficacy. On the other hand, if this psychoanalytic practitioner decides that it is nearly impossible to change the diagnostic and treatment style in the middle of a career, then the practitioner has failed to demonstrate self-efficacy. **Self-efficacy is an incredibly powerful tool to assist practitioners who are faced with tremendous change like that currently being experienced in the behavioral health care industry.** Assuming this same practitioner has a clear mental image of what success looks like in this new world of mental health care delivery, demonstrates the self-efficacy with respect to short-term therapy, then it becomes critical that others in the environment model the desired performance behaviors and create an environment that makes it easy for this psychoanalytic practitioner to practice short-term therapy. The essential components of this model are as follows: person, symbolic processes, self-control, behavior, modeling, and environment. Figure 1 shows the interrelationships of this social learning theory model.

Description

The PMS model is a five-phase model designed to maximize performance at all these levels simultaneously: task, position, team, department, division, and organization. **In many organizations performance is maximized at one level but results in a decline of performance in another valued area.** An illustrative example is a performance requirement to increase collections on delinquent patient accounts resulting in a mandate for practitioners to ask for payment at the end of the therapeutic encounter. This push for payment on delinquent accounts may result in an increase in collections and a reduction in account receivable days. An unintended consequence, however, might be a decrease in referrals from patients themselves and poor ratings on patient satisfaction instruments, not to mention provider satisfaction tools.

Managing performance represents managing a web of relationships, dependencies, goals, and consequences rather than focusing on one area of performance to the exclusion of other areas. In short, performance targets at all levels and throughout the organization must be aligned. These interdependencies represent the nature of the behavior of interactive systems. Not only is PMS an interactive system, but it is also organized into five iterative phases, as depicted in table 7.

This five-phase model is also developmental in that each phase builds upon and reinforces the preceding phase. The goal of PMS is to clearly set job-related behaviors at a defined point in time and to monitor each employee over a wide sampling of performance behaviors in order for each employee to achieve his or her full potential and fully contribute to the goals of the organization. Table 7 describes each phase in greater detail.

Reward and Recognition Function: Compensation, Benefits, and Communication

Reward and recognition is typically regarded as fluff. Specifically, compensation and benefits are seen as necessary evils. This line of logic stems from an organizational preoccupation with fulfilling legal requirements rather than investing in the potential and contribution of employees. In

TABLE 7. Phases of Performance Management System (PMS)

Phase	Description
Expectations	Set behaviorally based expectations for a specified time period
Development	Provide the necessary orientation, training, and experiences to create a performance-enhancing environment
Coaching	Offer regular, developmental feedback out of concern for the employee as a person and as a way of maximizing their full potential
Refining	Give behaviorally specific feedback based upon mutual problem solving around performance enhancement
Reporting	Document in a legally defensible, timely, fair, and understandable manner the performance behaviors that are on-target, approximating target, and off-target along with recommendations for improvement

most organizations accountants record employees as costs and/or liabilities. This accounting practice results in employees being viewed as expenditures to be reduced or costs to be contained rather than as precious resources that have unbounded potential if the proper investment is made to unleash this potential and target the potential in the direction of contributing to the organization.

More than any other function, reward and recognition is the most challenging. Fundamentally, managing the reward and recognition function is akin to managing paradox. The classic paradox is framed in the following question: **How does an organization invest (or spend) the minimum amount in resources (compensation and benefits) in order to get a maximum return on the investment (or justify the expenditure)?** The stated bias of this chapter is to view the reward and recognition function as an investment rather than as a cost or liability. These two views are contrasted in table 8.

Again, an investment in employees can yield returns on employee satisfaction, patient satisfaction, outcomes, and even profitability. An effective reward and recognition system consists of these three elements: compensation, benefits, and communication.

Compensation

Compensation refers to the financial payments earned by employees in exchange for services performed. The familiar adage "You Get What You Pay For" is as applicable in employment settings as it is in consumer settings. Do not expect to obtain Nordstrom service and Saks Fifth Avenue quality at Walmart prices. Similarly, do not expect to obtain stellar performance and superb customer service at minimum wage salaries. **You get what you pay for.**

Pfeffer (1998) warns leaders and managers of organizations designing compensation schemes to avoid the following six dangerous myths about pay: (1) equating labor rates and labor costs; (2) decreasing labor costs

TABLE 8. Contrasting Views of Reward and Recognition

Cost Perspective	Investment Perspective
Organizational liability	Organizational asset
Efficiency focused	Effectiveness focused
Emphasizes resources	Emphasizes outcomes
Current production	Current and future production
Justify expenditures	Maximize Return on Investment (ROI)
Replace with lower cost producer	Fully develop potential of current producer

solely but cutting labor rates; (3) assuming that a significant proportion of total costs consist of labor costs; (4) believing that low labor costs represent a source of competitive advantage; (5) expecting that individual incentive pay improves performance at the group and organization level; and (6) operating as if employees work only for money. These six dangerous myths should be avoided.

Compensation is commonly divided into direct and indirect pay. Direct pay includes the following types of pay: salary (exempt employees), hourly rate (nonexempt employees), bonuses, incentives, and stock options in some cases. Indirect pay includes the following: vacation time, holiday time, sick time, benefits, and discounts. Employees tend to value direct pay more than indirect pay. Yet many employees value direct and indirect pay for different reasons. Employers, in contrast, value both direct and indirect pay because the sum of the two types of pay equals total cash compensation.

Compensation is one of the more frequently heard complaints in mental health care organizations. The complaints range from the inadequacy of compensation to inequity in the pay structure. Employers determine the rate of pay for each position and also the relative attractiveness of the compensation of the entire organization in comparison to the local labor market. The compensation level of the firm in comparison to the labor market is derived from the compensation philosophy of the organization.

There exist three distinct compensation philosophies. They are as follows: lead market, meet market, and lag market. The respective compensation philosophy of the organization is determined by the executive team in consultation with in-house compensation expertise and compensation consulting firms. The lead market philosophy places a premium on wages and seeks to attract and retain employees based upon above-market wages. This is often known as the "Golden Hand Cuffs" approach to compensation. The meet market philosophy places a premium on reflecting the mean or median market wages. The lag market philosophy places a premium on nonfinancial mechanisms to attract and retain employees. For instance, organizations that are internationally renowned can afford to offer below-market wages due to the fact that there are more candidates wanting to become affiliated with an organization that is world famous. The Menninger Clinic and the World Health Organization are examples of organizations that can afford to compensate employees below market.

The determination of a compensation philosophy represents the starting point for most organizations. The next compensation decision is to determine the number of grades, steps, or levels of compensation. Organizations that have few levels are regarded as flat organizations. There are some advantages and disadvantages to flat organizations. The advantages are faster response time, less bureaucracy, clearer communication, and decreased number of hand-offs. The disadvantages of a flat organization are less opportunities for promotion, increased responsibility, and decision making pushed further down the organization. Employees typically value a structured career progression along with corresponding increases in compensation. Thus, employees prefer organizations that have a greater number of levels if compensation is associated with climbing the ladder. In contrast, more and more organizations are uncoupling compensation increases from climbing the ladder to performing. As such, pay-for-performance plans are increasing in frequency.

Pay-for-performance plans are not the same as merit-based pay. Merit-based pay is common to most mental health organizations. Merit-based pay provides employees with an annual increase in pay based upon the rated performance of the employee. In theory highly rated employees receive higher merit increases. Most mental health care organizations, however, place a ceiling on the percentage increase that is built into the merit increase pool. The percentage increase of most merit pools is closely associated with the inflation rate. Hence, if the inflation rate is 2.4 percent, then it would not be unusual that the maximum merit increase to be given to the most highly appraised employee would be 3.0 percent. If the maximum is 3.0 percent and the minimum percentage increase for employees not meeting expectations is 0 percent, then a critical question to be addressed is as follows: Is 3.0 percent a sufficient difference to motivate employees to perform well above expectations when employees that are performing well below expectations receive 0 percent and employees that are simply meeting expectations might receive 1.5 percent? **The motivational and organizational justice aspects of compensation cannot be underestimated.**

Compensation has been used by a host of companies to motivate employees to accomplish individual tasks in the achievement of organizational goals. The application of reinforcement theory is critical in the design of a motivating compensation scheme. Behaviorists tell us that intermittent feedback provides the greatest degree of motivational strength and regularly scheduled feedback provides the least degree of motivational strength. As such, incentive compensation that is received intermittently and not tied to any specific quantity factor provides the greatest motivational strength. In stark contrast, the regularly scheduled paycheck, whether once a week or twice a month, provides the least motivational strength. In fact, practitioners with a great deal of managerial experience realize that simply paying employees to do their jobs is often insufficient for employees to actually do their jobs not to mention exceed performance expectations. Many practitioners fantasize about working with a clinical population that is introspective, insightful, highly verbal, and intrinsically motivated. Mental health executives and managers share a similar fantasy with respect to their employees.

Compensation as stated earlier becomes a symbol of justice in the eyes of employees. Equity theory equips mental health executives and managers with a theoretical model to devise compensation schemes that are perceived as fair by employees. According to equity theory, an employee who feels that they are overworked and underpaid is predicted to do two things to achieve equity: ask for an increase in pay or decrease work load. Employees factor their input into the equity equation as well as the input of other workers. Specifically, an employee may feel that they are paid a fair wage until they discover that a coworker who came on board one year after they did in the same position is receiving 10 percent more in income. Similar to the other employee who feels overworked and underpaid, this employee will attempt to balance the scales of compensation justice. What can mental health care executives and managers do to prevent this from occurring? First, all employees should be educated about how compensation schemes are determined in their organization. Second, all employees should be informed about the external labor market and how price or salary sensitive the market happens to be depending upon the labor supply and labor demand for specific positions. Third, all employees should know the total cash value of both direct and indirect pay. Fourth, and most important, all employees should be compensated financially and psychosocially, as suggested in the chapter on organization behavior.

Benefits

Dolan (1998) asserts that **the design and administration of a benefit plan represents a source of competitive advantage with respect to recruiting and retaining high-performing practitioners.** Benefits include an increasingly diverse set of offerings. Typical benefits provided to employees include the following: health insurance, disability insurance, life insurance, pension plans, and many others. The design of a benefits plan should be based upon two technologies. First, employees should be viewed as customers of the organization and all of the concepts described in the chapter on marketing can be easily applied to employees in the design of a benefits package that meets the needs and wants of employees. Second, practitioners trained in life span development will suggest that during different development periods that basic needs change in order to meet the developmental milestones of that period. Accordingly, benefits should also be designed from a life span developmental perspective.

An emerging dilemma on the horizon is the fact that millions of baby boomer practitioners have underfunded their retirement plan contributions as organizations have moved away from defined-contribution pension plans to 403(b), 401(k), and other self-directed pension plans. It is very important for the welfare of baby boomer practitioners and the generation behind the baby boomers that organizations provide financial education to all employees in order to maximize contributions to pension plans based upon empirically tested guidelines regarding risk and other investment principles. Farber (1998) provides a summary of the basic lesson to be learned when providing financial education for employees: **Put in as much as you can as soon as you can for as long as you can.**

Communication

Communication is the essence of reward and recognition in organizations. Employees need to know by the behaviors that managers display that they are valued, cared for, respected, and, some would even argue, liked. Employees that experience caring and compassion as persons not just employees typically will perform at higher levels than those employees that experience an environment in which they view themselves as simply units of productivity. This is particularly true among mental health practitioners. Most individuals attracted to mental health as a profession are sensitive to interpersonal dynamics and the degree of caring and compassion that characterizes the culture and climate of the organization.

Legal/Regulatory Function: Minimizing Risk Exposure

There is a furious debate in the halls of government and the corridors of mental health organizations. There are many that feel that the federal and state government have gone too far in protecting the rights of employees due to the seemingly ever-increasing number and scope of employment and labor laws. On the other hand, there are many who believe that there are not enough laws and/or not enough enforcement resources to adequately protect the rights of employees. Both sides are probably right. The focus of this section, however, will be on the historical development of employment and labor laws in the United States and a basic understanding of the major employment and labor laws of importance to practitioners functioning in managerial or supervisory roles.

The historical development of employment and labor law in this nation parallels the history of the United States. In general, the United States does not favor government involvement and perceived intrusion in the matters of individual and corporate concern. Yet the U.S. Constitution, subject to interpretation as determined by the U.S. Supreme Court, and State Constitutions, subject to interpretation by State Supreme Courts, clearly outline legal principles that protect the safety, health, and welfare of all U.S. citizens. **Hence, the basis of employment and labor law in the United States is to protect the safety, health, and welfare of all U.S. citizens who are engaged in work in this country or work in another country for a U.S.-owned company.**

Occupational social workers, occupational health psychologists, occupational nurses, and occupational psychiatrists are well aware of the dangers facing employees at work. In fact, the National Institutes for Occupational Safety and Health (NIOSH) studies the incidence and prevalence of occupational diseases and injuries. However, dangers at work are not limited to disease, injury, and illness. Other dangers include pay inequity, sexual harassment, racial harassment, humiliation, and a host of other acts committed by managers, supervisors, and coworkers and often not challenged by employers. As we approach the twenty-first century, new dangers are on the horizon. One of the more noteworthy dangers is the gradual erosion of job security in the form of layoffs. An all-too-common scenario is as follows:

> A fifty-three-year-old practitioner is having a conversation with several other practitioners over the age of fifty and they discover much to their chagrin that they have been the victims of the corporate downsizing at their HMO. The executives of the HMO stated that the downsizing was a strategic response to market share and financial pressures and that a rigorous layoff selection process based on performance was used to determine who would remain on staff and who would receive a notice of layoff. These fifty-plus practitioners are suspect. In fact, out of a total of twenty practitioners and managers, each and every one who was laid off was over the age of fifty.

What legal protection exits for these fifty-plus-year-old practitioners and managers? There is an act that was passed by Congress to protect workers over the age of forty from being not laid off but cast off corporate ships into the violent waves of corporate tropical storms. This federal act is called the Age Discrimination in Employment Act (ADEA). This act was drafted to protect the employment rights of all workers over the age of forty. What is magical about the age of forty? It was discovered that workers over the age of forty were often targets of layoffs and targets of termination several years prior to receiving lifetime retirement benefits. Also, there still exists an age bias toward workers over the age of forty, although a host of empirical data suggests that most of these stereotypes are simply biases and nothing more.

Table 9 highlights the major federal employment and labor laws that practitioners need to be aware of both as a manager and supervisor and as an employee of a mental health organization. Many of these laws apply to organizations of a certain size in terms of the number of employees.

It is critically important to consult with an appropriately trained attorney specializing in employment and labor law prior to all situations that involve legal issues. Unfortunately, the management of human resources has become an increasingly risky area for organizations, managers, and even practitioners. Risk management and prevention are one and the same.

TABLE 9. Major Federal Employment and Labor Laws

Law	Year	Description
Wagner Act	1935	Legally defined unions and established National Labor Relations Board
Fair Labor Standards Act	1938	Minimum wage, overtime pay, and child labor laws established
Equal Pay Act	1963	Prohibits unequal pay for same job. Intent was to equalize pay for men and women in the same job
Title VII of Civil Rights Act	1964	Prohibits discrimination based upon color, national origin, race, religion, and sex in **all** employment-related decisions
Executive Order 11246	1965	Requires affirmative action for certain organizations only
Age Discrimination in Employment Act	1967	Prohibits discrimination among employees forty or older in **all** employment-related decisions
Occupational Safety and Health Act	1970	Prohibits the harm of employees by establishing safety and health standards
Pregnancy Discrimination Act	1978	Prohibits discrimination against pregnant women
Immigration Reform and Control Act	1986	Prohibits discrimination against workers based upon citizenship status
Worker Adjustment and Retraining Act	1988	Prohibits organizations from laying off employees without notification in certain cases
American with Disabilities Act	1990	Prohibits discrimination based upon disability status
Civil Rights Act	1991	Prohibits quotas and allows punitive damages
Family and Medical Leave Act	1994	Unpaid leave required for "serious health conditions" and family matters like childbirth, adoption, and caring for an ill relative

Retrenchment Function

An increasing number of organizations, including mental health organizations, are painfully deciding to retrench, pull back, and downsize. This trend that began in the 1980s is forecasted to continue well into the twenty-first century according to many academics and labor experts. **In fact, the term *lay-off* may very well be a misnomer now because, unlike in the past, most workers who are laid off today never return to work for the same employer.** A more appropriate term to describe the reality of downsizing today is *cast off.* Employees today are literally thrown overboard into the stormy seas of corporate tropical depressions.

The depression does not stop at the doors of the organization that has either strategically decided to retrench or in the case of most organizations had to quickly react to a market force or financial pressure that caught the organization by surprise. The physiological and psychological toll on employees but particularly highly skilled professionals and managers is very high when faced with the reality that their employment has been terminated (Cobb, Brooks, Kasl, and Connely 1966; Kaufmann 1981).

The puzzling phenomenon that occurs in organizations that downsize is that quite often the cost savings and financial returns targeted to be achieved as a result of the downsizing do not occur. Cascio, Young, and Morris (1997) discovered in a sample of 5,479 organizations, in a period between 1980 and 1994, that there was not a statistically significant difference between organizations that downsized and those that did not with respect to higher financial returns. How can this be? Several factors emerge that account for this financial fact. First, in most cases job, work, and process design does not accompany the reduction in the number of employees. Hence, the workload remains the same, but there are fewer workers to do the work, and over time those remaining workers become ineffective, inefficient, and/or burn out. Second, far too many organizations focus on only the laid-off employees and not the survivors or even the managers that were given the dreaded task of deciding who the organization would retain and then communicating to an employee that their employment relationship was over. Survivors and many managers involved in the decision-making and communication process are full of a wide range of emotions that interfere with optimal performance and productivity on the job. Third, the more competent and confident practitioners, realizing that organizations typically do not downsize only once, become concerned, anxious, and begin their job search in another work setting. As such, the intellectual capital walks out the door. Fourth, practitioners are shaken by the frightening reality that security does not rest in the hands of the employer but in the hands of each practitioner. In other words, the psychological contract is fundamentally and radically altered when an organization downsizes.

Eby and Bush (1998) recommend that employers provide advance notice, communicate honestly, openly, and often, and implement support services. It is absolutely essential that the mental health care organization that downsizes implement the aforementioned recommendations to prevent poor financial returns, slipping market share, tumbling employee satisfaction, and declining patient satisfaction and quality of care. There are costs associated with designing and implementing these recommendations. Yet these costs must be viewed as a wise investment to prevent the "dumbsizing" of the workforce (Baumohl 1993). *Dumbsizing* refers to all of the intended and unintended negative consequences of downsizing as described in the previous paragraph.

Discipline Function

The disciplinary function is a necessary evil in all organizations including mental health organizations. There comes a time when employees will simply not respond to interventions designed to enhance their performance without the imposition of sanctions. **Discipline should be conducted from a caring and compassionate perspective rather than as a punitive maneuver designed to hurt, humiliate, and destroy.** Most organizations have a discipline policy to assist managers in the proper and legally defensible approach to enhancing the performance of employees by imposing certain work-related sanctions.

Unfortunately, employers and mental health administrators are confronted with situations that are not amenable to change using coaching, development, feedback, or training in those cases in which a mental health practitioner has knowingly violated a norm, policy, procedure, or standard and even a law. The keyword is *knowingly.* Administrators should not hold practitioners accountable for behaviors that they were not aware violated a norm, policy, procedure, or law. Thus, this places a burden on supervisors to orient, educate, and train practitioners well to prevent the practitioner from claiming that they did not know. There are certain behaviors, like spitting, however, that clearly do not have to spelled out in an orientation program for a practitioner to know that this behavior is unacceptable in any health care work setting.

It is critical that practitioners receive a copy of the organization's code of conduct, standards of performance, and appropriate policy and procedures manuals and that the practitioner sign in writing indicating that they understand and agree to abide by all of the aforementioned documents. Furthermore, it is essential that a discipline policy be shared with each practitioner and that they sign a document indicating that they are aware of the policy and procedures for disciplining employees. This set of exchanges between the organization and the practitioner fall under the umbrella of minimizing liability for both parties and establishing due process.

In the unlikely event that a practitioner should knowingly violate a norm, standard, policy, procedure, or law, then it is incumbent upon the supervisor to follow the discipline policies and procedures designed by the organization. This establishes due process. Failure to abide by the discipline policies, procedures, and past practice robs the practitioner facing the discipline charge without due process. In all cases documentation is absolutely essential without exception. If conflict escalates and the issue becomes a legal situation resulting in a jury trial, then it must be noted that juries have the opportunity to study written testimony while deliberating but have to recall verbal testimony while deliberating. Mental health practitioners know the limitations of recall as a memory strategy and the importance of cues as a memory enhancer.

A growing number of organizations including health care organizations are implementing positive discipline programs. **Positive discipline is not an oxymoron.** The goal of positive discipline is to provide the practitioner with the tools necessary and sufficient to succeed as a valued employee. The goal is not to catch the practitioner doing something wrong and then try them before their peers and, finally, symbolically hang them at the next multidisciplinary case conference. Most positive discipline programs are four-step processes. The steps are progressive. The steps move from informal and verbal warnings to formal, written warnings and, ultimately, to recommendation for involuntary termination. In some organizations the step prior to recommending involuntary termination allows practitioners time to reflect on their behavior and decide what actions they might want to take in light of the situation. This time period might be called "decision-making leave" or other names. The purpose of this time period, however, remains the same.

Many organizations also have a process for employees that have been found to be in violation of a norm, standard, policy, or procedure and have been formally sanctioned by the organization to appeal or grieve the matter. As such, organizations have written appeal and grievance policies and procedures. Again, one of the driving forces of these policies and procedures is to establish due process and communicate procedural fairness. Appeal and grievance processes typically depend upon the executive management of an organization to review the facts and then render a decision. In many cases the grieving practitioner will decide if they are dissatisfied with the outcome (distributive justice) that they will seek the counsel of an attorney or go to the press. As a result, an increasing number of organizations are implementing **Alternative Dispute Resolution (ADR) programs.**

A properly designed and implemented positive discipline program can minimize exposure to litigation. The adoption of an ADR program, however, can provide a little extra insurance. Ritzky (1997) estimates that litigation to settle employment disputes has grown 2,000 percent since the 1970s. The cost of defending employment dispute cases has mushroomed to a range of $75,000 to $100,000 today (Gallagher 1994). ADR is a cost-effective and cost-efficient way to address employment disputes.

ADR ranges from arbitration to voluntary mediation. ADR is increasingly being used by health care organizations (DeSouza 1998). The common theme among all the various types of ADR programs is the involvement of a neutral third party. In the case of arbitration the neutral third party hears all of the facts and then renders a decision. The decision may or may not be binding upon both parties. In the case of voluntary mediation the neutral third party creates an environment in which each party presents their case and is encouraged to listen and understand the other side and then move toward an agreement that satisfies both parties. **Mediators do not render decisions; mediators facilitate.** Mediation seems to be a worthwhile dispute resolution process for mental health organizations to consider given the fact that it is aligned with the values and norms of practitioners.

Labor Relations Function

There has always been a debate in the United States about the purpose and utility of unions. The history of unions parallels the history of commerce. During the agricultural era unions were virtually non-existent because most individuals worked for themselves or worked in a role as a sharecropper, indentured servant, and even a slave. During the industrial age more and more workers became employees of large factories that were governed by supervisors and managers who organized, planned, controlled, scheduled, and compensated the work of the employees. In many cases employees voiced their concerns to management regarding unsafe conditions, inadequate pay and benefits, and perceptions of unfair treatment. Some organizations responded to the voice of workers, while other organizations decided to ignore the voice of workers. As a result, unions proliferated during the industrial age. The explicit purpose of unions was to protect the safety, health, and welfare of employees. Today, during the service era, unions are dying out in some industries and growing in others. Health care organizations represent a growing area for unions.

The rise of managed health care has resulted in an increasing number of practitioners who are voicing their concerns for the safety, health, and welfare of the practitioner and patient community. Astute organizations are listening and responding. Other organizations are ignoring and even defending their positions. As such, a growing number of practitioners are turning to unions to represent their interests and attempt through the collective bargaining process to mandate that organizations adopt policies, procedures, and practices that protect the safety, health, and welfare of both practitioners and patients. **Even physicians are organizing.**

The National Labor Relations Board, which governs disputes between management and labor, ruled that salaried physicians could organize because they did not act in a supervisory capacity (Lowes 1998). The keyword is *salaried.* This presents a problem for union organizers. The bulk of practitioners are not employees but owners and independent contractors. Current law governing unions excludes owners and independent contractors from joining unions. Yet some members of Congress are contemplating introducing legislation that might challenge this age-old requirement in light of the new realities of the service economy.

Managers of mental health care organizations who desire to prevent practitioners from joining unions should follow some simple yet sound advice. **Treat practitioners the way that they would like to be treated with respect to safety, health, welfare, and fairness.** Union avoidance boils down to designing and operating mental health care organizations that fully utilize the potential of all practitioners in such a way that practitioners are excited and energized about fully contributing to the goals of the organization. In short, **do the right thing, even if it costs you a little bit of money and time.**

Conclusion

All types of organizations are struggling to acquire and sustain a competitive advantage. Mental health care organizations are no exception. Behavioral health care technology is largely shared among competing mental health organizations, the range of legal business structures is limited by federal and state laws, and the skills and qualifications of mental health personnel are largely determined by accreditation, licensing, and credentialing bodies. As such, one of the only resources that any mental health care organization can leverage is the human resources of the organization.

Some factors that differentiate between one mental health care organization and another include the way in which the employees utilize the behavioral health technology, the manner in which deals are constructed given the framework established by federal and state laws, and the continuous development of capacities at the level of the individual practitioner, at the level of the team, and at the level of the mental health organization. Ulrich (1998) argues that human resources can provide a foundation for organizational excellence by focusing on both the strategic and operational linkages among human resources and the other organizational functions as well as enabling human resources to provide the expertise necessary to transform a stable, static mental health care organization into a learning organization.

In essence, the role of any mental health administrator during these times of turbulent change and opportunity is similar to the role of a conductor. The conduct of an orchestra communicates expectations, makes certain that all of the players know their role and their responsibilities, reads from the same musical score as the players, and then carefully observes and makes changes to bring the musical score to life based upon a dynamic exchange of energy among the conductor, the orchestra, and the audience. All of this translates into an enjoyable and memorable experience. Mental health care organizations are more than simply providers of a service. Mental health care organizations are framers of an experience that enables patients and their families to feel compassion, wholeness, and completeness.

GLOSSARY

Affirmative action Legal concept and set of policies and procedures enforced by the Equal Employment Opportunity Commission (EEOC) to treat protected groups of employees affirmatively to remedy past and current discriminatory practices

Arbitration One of the methods of Alternative Dispute Resolution (ADR) in which a third-party neutral renders a decision on a case involving conflict between two or more employees or between management and labor

Bargaining unit Group of two or more employees who share common interests with respect to working conditions and collectively bargain for the improvement or the maintenance of a prescribed set of working conditions

Career paths Systematic and developmental lines of vertical or horizontal advancement within a given organization

Cutoff score Bottom-line score that a candidate is required to meet in order to make a wide range of employment decisions such as hiring, firing, and even, considering an employee for training

Discipline A process that is established by a policy and governed by a set of procedures that attempts to improve work-related performance by establishing legally defensible sanctions

Due process The right of an employee to be treated in a way that is spelled out in the organization's policies and procedures

Equity theory A theory of motivation in which employees compare themselves to others with regard to work output and compensation

Exempt Category of employees that are not covered by the Fair Labor Standards Act with respect to overtime compensation

Feedback A process of communication in which one employee provides information about a work-related behavior with the goal of attempting to enhance the performance of that employee

Golden handcuffs A compensation approach in which employees are paid at above-market wages in order to encourage retention

Grievance A formal policy and procedure that governs disputes between labor and management

Job grade Payment structure for positions in which each job is assigned a grade that determines the rate of pay

Job posting and bidding Internal announcement of a vacancy within an organization

Labor market Refers to the geographic, industrial, and/or occupational area from which candidates are drawn to be considered for employment

Labor relations A set of policies and procedures to guide the organization in effective and legal ways to manage the relationship between labor and management

Mediation One of the methods of ADR in which a third-party neutral intervenes in dispute between two or more employees but allows the employees to make a mutually agreeable decision regarding the dispute

Merit-based pay Set of policies and procedures dictating how merit pay should be allocated

Nonexempt Category of employees covered by the Fair Labor Standards Act who are paid one and one-half times their usual rate if they work over the standard work week

Organizational development A technology used to enhance the functioning of organizations

Orientation A formal process to socialize new employees to the organization and the job

Pay-for-performance A compensation method that attempts to link compensation with set standards of performance

Progressive discipline A method to discipline employees that represents a multi-step process ranging from an informal conversation to a recommendation for termination

Recognition A tool used by employers to acknowledge employees formally for work well done

Recruitment Process by which employers increase awareness of the organization and certain employment vacancies to candidates

Reward A tool used by employers to reinforce employees formally for achieving a designated performance standard

Selection Process by which employers make a decision about which candidate to hire for a certain position

Sexual harassment Set of policies and procedures to protect members of both sexes from experiencing a hostile work environment and bargaining based upon gender

Socialization Process by which employees learn about the culture, values, and climate of an organization and department

Training A system developed by the employer to provide employees with the knowledge, skills, and experiences necessary to perform well in their current roles and in their future roles

Wage Total cash compensation including salary and benefits

REFERENCES

Baumohl, B. 1993. When downsizing becomes "dumbsizing." *Time,* 15 March, 55.

Cobb, S., G. W. Brooks, S. V. Kasl, and W. E. Connely. 1966. The health of people changing jobs: A description of a longitudinal study. *American Journal of Public Health* 56:1476–81.

Day, N. 1998. Informal learning gets results. *Workforce* 77:31–36.

DeSouza, J. R. 1998. ADR: Methods of addressing workplace conflict in health services organizations. *Journal of Healthcare Management* 43:453–67.

Dolan, K. P. 1998. Fringes: The wider choices, the happier the staff. *Medical Economics,* 12 January, 117–27.

Farber, L. 1998. Keeping close tabs on your retirement plan. *Medical Economics,* 13 July, 150–60.

Gallagher, M. M. 1994. ADR slices litigation cost, enhances morale. *HR Focus* 71:19–20.

Ganzel, R. 1998. Putting out the welcome mat. *Training* 35:54–62.

Gazier, K. L. 1998. Managing behavioral health. *Journal of Healthcare Management* 43:393–96.

Kaipa, P., C. Newham, and R. Volckmann. 1998. Aligning strategy, processes, and people through pyramid building. *Systems Thinker* 9:1–5.

Kaufman, H. 1981. *Professionals in Search of Work: Coping with Stress of Job Loss and Underemployment.* New York: Interscience.

Lowes, R. L. 1998. Strength in numbers: Could doctor unions really be the answer? *Medical Economics* 115–24.

Pfeffer, J. 1998. Six dangerous myths about pay. *Harvard Business Review* 76:109–19.

Richards, S. C. 1985. Work and study problems. In M. Hersen and A. S. Bellack, eds., *Handbook of Clinical Behavior Therapy with Adults.* New York: Plenum Press.

Ritzky, A. A. 1997. Employment litigation hits the big leagues. *Best Reviews–Property–Casualty Insurance Edition* (February): 86–87.

Rosenbluth, H. F., and D. M. Peters. 1998. *Good Company: Caring as Fiercely as You Compete.* Reading, MA: Addison-Wesley.

Senge, P. 1990. *The Fifth Discipline: The Art and Practice of The Learning Organization.* New York: Doubleday Currency.

Ulrich, D. 1998. A new mandate for human resources. *Harvard Business Review* 76:124–34.

CHAPTER 10

Outcomes Assessment and Performance Improvement: Measurements and Methodologies That Matter in Mental Health Care

Marie A. Krousel-Wood, M.D., M.S.P.H.

Measuring what matters in medicine is gaining popularity in the current era of accountability in health care. With the unrelenting focus on medical costs and how to contain them, there is growing concern about the preservation of the quality of clinical practice. Evaluating clinical practice through the measurement of clinical performance and clinical outcomes is becoming increasingly important. In fact, it is mandated by many agencies that accredit health care organizations. **The most challenging decision for administrators and others is deciding what and how to measure variables that actually assess the quality of clinical practice.**

Defining quality in mental health care (and health care in general) is often difficult. Nevertheless, quality in health care ultimately rests with patient outcomes (Chowanec 1994; 1996). Understanding the links between patient outcomes and what we do in medicine (processes) provides a framework for continuous quality/performance improvement—a concept that focuses on improving poor outcomes or maximizing good outcomes through appropriate changes to the processes of care (Chowanec 1996; Srebnik et al. 1997).

Although the core principles of outcomes assessment (OA) and continuous quality/performance improvement are related, the application of these principles are varied and numerous. Outcomes data is being used for internal (i.e., institution-specific performance improvement activities), external (i.e., public accountability), and research purposes. In this essay core principles will be outlined and examples provided to illustrate key points. The strategies and approaches described can be applied to various clinical and management scenarios. The objectives of this chapter are as follows: (1) define and discuss health care outcomes: what are outcomes? who is measuring outcomes? why measure outcomes? where is outcomes data? (2) describe the multifaceted approach to outcomes assessment and performance improvement; and (3) identify benefits of and barriers to outcomes assessment and performance improvement.

Objective 1: Define and Describe Health Care Outcomes

What Are Outcomes?

Health care outcomes are measures of the end result of what happens to patients as a consequence of their encounter(s) with the health care system. The assessment of outcomes for groups of patients is an application of clinical epidemiology: the study of the distribution of disease in human populations and of the determinants that influence this disease distribution (Gordis 1996). **It is by looking at groups of patients (populations) that patterns emerge and trends are identified regarding treatment effectiveness and clinical outcomes.** This information may lead to improvements in health care delivery and ultimately health care outcomes in individual and groups of patients.

Outcomes are primarily classified in six different categories: mortality/survival, morbidity/clinical endpoints, functional status, pain, satisfaction, and cost (table 1). Dr. Donebedian grouped these into the *D*s of outcomes: **death, disease, disability, discomfort,** and **dissatisfaction.** More recently, **dollars** and **derangement** have been added to the list. Many current terms used reflect a broader focus regarding outcomes: survival, health promotion and disease prevention, functional ability, pain-free status, satisfaction, cost-effectiveness, and cost-benefit. Although the number of categories listed here are relatively few, the number of outcomes measures developed/identified to date are abundant. For example, the CONQUEST (Computerized Needs Oriented Quality Measurement Evaluation System) database contains information on approximately twelve hundred clinical performance (includes outcomes) measures that were developed by public and private organizations (see Internet site www.ahcpr.gov/qual/conquest.htm). Several of these measures are directly related to mental health: average number of patients reporting a remission for depression; change in functional limitations for patients with depression; inpatient complications for depressed elderly patients; and unsafe use of restraints for psychiatric patients. This database, although comprehensive and inclusive of different disease systems, is incomplete. Many groups and organizations (such as the Agency for Health Care Policy and Research [AHCPR] and the National Institute of Mental Health [NIMH]) have developed and continue to develop additional outcomes measures.

In relation to the medical care delivered, outcomes may be immediate or short term (e.g., in-hospital mortality for substance abuse patients), intermediate (e.g., one-year follow-up functional status post day treatment for depressed patients), or long term (e.g., five-year recidivism rate for schizophrenic patients). **The intermediate and long-term outcomes may be costly or difficult to obtain and temporally removed from the encounter of interest. As a result, process measures (what we do in medicine) are sometimes collected and reported as "surrogate outcomes" measures. This has been an acceptable alternative provided that the process surrogate outcome measure is closely related to the true outcome of interest.** For example, the actual costs for one year of treatment for depression may be difficult to obtain. Using claims data, however, the utilization of services (a surrogate for cost) by the depressed patients could be monitored: admissions/readmissions to the hospital / emergency room / day treatment unit; prescriptions filled for antidepressant or other medication; and number of

TABLE 1. Outcomes Categorization Examples

Mortality/Survival
In-hospital mortality
Five-year survival
Morbidity
Complications
Recidivism
Side effects
Functional Status
Physical functioning
Mental functioning
Role functioning
Pain
Pain index
Satisfaction
Overall satisfaction
Satisfaction with quality of care
Satisfaction with amenities of care
Cost
Cost-effectiveness
Cost-benefit
Resource utilization

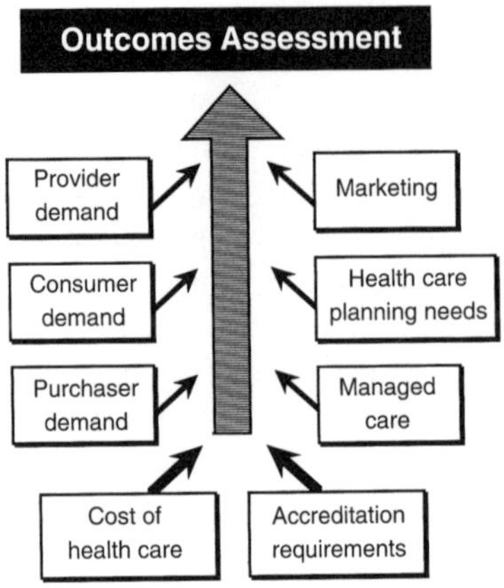
Outcomes Assessment
Provider demand
Consumer demand
Purchaser demand
Cost of health care
Accreditation requirements
Managed care
Health care planning needs
Marketing

Fig. 1. Drivers for outcomes assessment

clinic visits. Tracking the utilization of multiple services (process measures) by depressed patients in the one year follow-up period provides a basis for cost (outcome of interest) estimated during that time period.

Why Measure Outcomes?

The driving forces for the measurement of outcomes are numerous (fig. 1). In fact, many of the reasons are not new. Health care providers have long been interested in monitoring how well their patients do after a given treatment (Codman 1914). There is limited evidence-based information for many of the current medical practices; randomized controlled trials (RCT) have not been performed that would demonstrate efficacy (how well a treatment works under ideal circumstances for selected patients) for many technologies and treatments in use today. Monitoring outcomes for groups of patients over time has provided valuable information regarding treatment effectiveness (how well a treatment works under usual circumstances for patients in general) and quality of care. More recently, information has been published regarding variation in practice and outcomes (Wennberg 1998). Although certain variation in health care is considered good, inappropriate variation that can lead to poor outcomes is not desirable. Although RCTs are still considered the "gold standard" for determining treatment efficacy, observational outcomes studies are in essence natural experiments that provide information regarding what works under usual conditions in different patient groups.

Another driving force for outcomes measurement is the concern with the costs of medical care. As costs continue to be an issue in health care delivery (and in particular mental health care delivery), patients, providers, and purchasers want information that outcomes are good and quality of life is enhanced or maintained. In medicine we often perceive that doing something is better than doing nothing and that doing more is better than doing less. Outcomes assessment and analysis provides a framework for addressing this perception and subsequently proving or disproving the hypothesis for different clinical scenarios.

The penetration of managed care in the health care market has resulted in increased attention on population assessment, disease management programs for groups of patients with selected disorders and outcomes monitoring. These efforts are in large part driven by the requirements of accreditation organizations; however, they are also important in decision making for managed care administrators. **In order to maximize the health of the populations they serve, managed care organizations' (MCO) administrators must have information on the health status of their members. Outcomes assessment and monitoring provides such information.**

Who's Measuring Outcomes?

Those interested in collecting outcomes data can be categorized in one of three groups based on the primary use of the data: internal (institution-specific), external (public accountability), and research. The purpose for, use of, and extensiveness of collection of the outcomes information may vary depending on the group.

Internal groups include health care providers and administrators who use outcomes information to improve patient care and facilitate medical decision making. This data can also be used in the selection of health care technologies within an organization. In the realm of institution-specific performance improvement activities, outcomes measurement and monitoring provide the feedback necessary for management of the activities. Regarding an institution's use of clinical practice guidelines (provided they are appropriately used), outcomes data facilitates their development, refinement, and evaluation over time.

External groups include consumer organizations, purchasers (including the federal government), state and public health agencies, contract, and accreditation organizations. The primary goal of these entities is to assess/ensure public accountability of health care delivery systems in the United States. The Foundation for Accountability (FACCT) is a not-for-profit organization that brings together consumer groups and purchasers with the goal of helping Americans make better decisions in health care (www.facct.org). Although they target different diseases, they have outlined quality outcome measures for Major Depressive Disorder that include lost to follow-up, patient satisfaction, patient functional status, remittance, and patient ability to maintain daily activities. Under development are quality measures for alcohol misuse and dependency. These and other consumer-focused quality measures are designed to support and encourage public education regarding health care quality (www.facct.org).

An example of an independent state agency that is responsible for addressing escalating costs in health care, ensuring health care quality, and increasing access for all citizens is the Pennsylvania Health Care Cost Containment Council (www.phc4.org). They publish a number of consumer-oriented and other reports, including the "Consumer Guide to Coronary Artery Bypass Graft Surgery" and "Drug-Related Inpatient Hospitalizations: A Five-Year Perspective (1991–1995)."

The reporting of outcomes and performance data are being required by organizations that accredit health care entities: the Joint Commission on Accreditation of Healthcare Organizations (JCAHO) and the National Committee for Quality Assurance (NCQA). JCAHO is an independent not-for-profit organization that evaluates and accredits health care organizations in the United States, including hospitals, health care networks, managed care organizations, behavioral health care systems, and other health care systems. Their accreditation process has evolved recently to include integration of performance measurement (Joint Commission 1996; Klegon 1997). Outcome and clinical performance indicators that can be submitted to JCAHO by health plans and networks for the accreditation process are listed in the National Library of Healthcare Indicators (Joint Commission 1997). There are process and outcomes measures listed for depression and chemical dependency. **These measures present opportunities for interested administrators to participate in collection of mental health process and outcomes measures that can be compared with other participating institutions. In addition, there is opportunity to develop other relevant indicators.**

More explicit requirements for outcomes and performance elements are from NCQA and the Health Plan Employer Data Information Set (HEDIS). NCQA is a not-for-profit organization that was established to accredit managed care organizations. In order to meet accreditation requirements, MCOs must demonstrate active participation in population-relevant performance improvement activities, one of which has to be behavioral health. Quantifiable outcomes or process measures must be identified, monitored, and analyzed (to determine if the improvement was clinically meaningful and/or statistically significant). Other process and outcomes monitoring are required as well (NCQA 1998). HEDIS was codeveloped by NCQA and representatives of employers and health plans and includes indicators for mental health and substance abuse. Although participation in HEDIS is voluntary, the following measures in mental health are in the reporting set for Commercial, Medicare, and/or Medicaid members according to the 1999 HEDIS 3.0 specifications (HEDIS 3.0 1998): (1) follow-up after hospitalization for mental illness; (2) antidepressant medication management (new in 1999); (3) mental health utilization; and (4) chemical dependency utilization. Additional mental health measures are in the testing phases. These are primarily process measures. Data submitted from participating plans are used to compare health plans and to generate national averages that are used as benchmarks that are external goals that institutions can strive toward or exceed with respect to outcomes and process measures. NCQA features Quality Compass—a national database of plan-specific performance information generated from submitted HEDIS data. In 1998 data was submitted for Quality Compass from nearly three hundred health plans nationwide. This database is intended to be a decision and management support tool (www.ncqa.org). The national averages reported from this database are used by various health plans and other organizations as reference and benchmark information. The Health Care Financing Administration (HCFA) has issued the interim standards for the Quality Improvement System for Managed Care (QISMC) for organizations contracting with Medicare and Medicaid. One domain of the standards is the "Quality Assessment and Performance Improvement" (QAPI) program. QAPI requires engagement in performance improvement activities that result in improvement in processes that are expected to positively impact health outcomes and patient satisfaction (Operational Policy Letter no. 72 1998; www.aahp.org). Although HCFA is allowing an implementation phase-in period, it is anticipated that improvement in processes and/or outcomes for selected conditions will be required around the year 2001.

There are numerous external groups that are promoting and/or requiring health care organizations' investment in process and/or outcome accountability measures. These measures are supposed to provide an objective assessment of where a health care organization stands with respect to the selected measures for designated conditions in certain patient populations. **It is important to note that these measures rarely take into account variations in patient comorbidity, severity of primary illness, and/or age. Mental health care administrators should interpret this comparative health data with caution.**

Research groups: Health Services Researchers have made significant strides in the last several years regarding development and validation of outcomes tools, measures, and models. In the mental health care area the leading provider of funds for extramural services research is the National Institute of Mental Health (NIMH). Although it has supported traditional areas of health services research, it is expanding its investment and commitment to services research (Norquist and Magruder 1998). NIMH is not the only provider of grant funds for services research in mental health. AHCPR collaborated with NIMH on the Schizophrenia PORT (Patient Outcomes Research Team) and the Depression Collaborative Study. Other collaborations have occurred with the Veterans Affairs Administration, Center for Disease Control and Prevention, and the World Health Organization, to name a few (Norquist and MaGruder 1998). Results of this and other health services research collaboration provide the information needed regarding validity and reliability of outcomes tools and methods. In addition, it gives us the information on what works for selected persons with a given disorder under usual and/or optimal conditions. An example of an organization that promotes the science behind outcomes assessment is the Medical Outcomes Trust. The Medical Outcomes Trust is a nonprofit, public service organization that was incorporated in 1992. Its goal is to achieve a global adoption of health care outcomes assessment by advancing the science and use of the health outcomes measures (www.outcomes-trust.org). Information regarding outcomes instruments, resources, and trust membership can be obtained from this organization.

Where Is Outcomes Data?

Medical Records: Outcomes data can be found in a variety of places. **The "gold standard" has been the patient medical record. Although this is an important source of information, it is not a complete record of all outcomes of interest.** Patient functional status and satisfaction with care are typically not recorded in the patient medical record. In addition, patients may seek care in multiple institutions resulting in an incomplete record at any one site of care. When using the medical record as a source of outcomes information, one should consider the following: the relevance of the data element to the study/project question, the readability of the record, the reliability of the abstraction (particularly if multiple reviewers are used), the validity of the elements abstracted, and the availability to all pertinent records. Because reliability and validity will be mentioned in subsequent sections of this chapter, further discussion regarding their definitions are warranted. Reliability refers to the accuracy and reproducibility of the data collected. Validity refers to the ability of a tool to measure what it purports to measure (Gordis 1996; Rothman 1986). To use a nonmedical example, let's say that an archer is engaged in target practice; the goal is to hit the bull's eye on target B. If after ten tries she consistently hits the bull's eye on target A, the hits would be accurate (she hit the bull's eye), reproducible (she hit the bull's eye consistently), but not valid (she hit the wrong target). **It is important in health care to have outcomes and process measures that are reliable and valid indicators of what actually happens in medical practice.**

Because we have not yet achieved a universal automated patient medical record, most medical records are manually kept and may be difficult to read. For those collecting outcomes data from this source, it would be beneficial to assign a physician or other over-reader in the event that the reviewer is unable to read the chart. This would enhance the reliability and validity of the abstracted data.

Surveys/Questionnaires: Outcomes data are also found in questionnaires or surveys from both patients and providers. Surveys are typically used when collecting information such as satisfaction with care, functional status (e.g., mental, physical, social), demographic information (such as education and income levels), pain index, and depression/anxiety scale. There are a number of important issues to consider when using surveys or interpreting data collected from surveys. The questionnaire should be readable (e.g., large, bold print with a simple font) and appropriate to the reading level for the population surveyed (e.g., an eighth-grade reading level is sometimes employed to meet the minimum standards for selected patients surveyed). In addition, the questions asked should be relevant to the study/project goals and should be feasible to complete in a given time period (e.g., lengthy surveys may not be completed). Questionnaires used to determine outcomes should undergo reliability and validity testing to ensure that the data collected is reproducible, accurate, and measures what it is supposed to measure (McDowell and Newel 1987).

Information Systems: Information systems are another primary source of outcomes data. In fact, the use of administrative or billing data is rapidly increasing because of the ready availability of this data through claims processing. Although administrative databases are widely available, there are disadvantages to their use: they do not collect clinical factors that are not diagnostic; they include a limited number of secondary diagnosis; and they are not able to distinguish between complications and comorbidities (Hannan et al. 1997). Therefore, it is important when using this data that one understand what the basis is for the data collection and storage. That is, what codes are used (International Classification of Diseases, Ninth Revision [ICD-9], Current Procedural Terminology, Fourth Revision [CPT-4], Diagnostic Related Groups [DRG]); whether primary and/or secondary diagnosis/procedure codes are available; the maximum/minimum number of codes allowed for submission/storage; the length of time the codes are stored; and the reimbursement rules. Another issue that relates to coding is the accuracy of the codes used in mental health. In an NCQA pilot study of HEDIS there was substantial disagreement between the medical record and the administrative data in measuring outpatient follow-up of patients hospitalized with major affective disorder (Epstein 1995). Also, reimbursement for mental health services and uncertainty of diagnosis have been reported to result in miscoding and incomplete coding of selected mental health conditions (Rost et al. 1994). For example, patients may not have a policy that covers hospitalization for substance abuse (e.g., alcoholism). The alcoholic patient may also be depressed and the hospitalization claim may only reflect depression as a reason for admission. If one were attempting to track outcomes for patients admitted for alcoholism, this incomplete coding would not include this patient in the data set. **If miscoding is a frequent occurrence, this could result in an underrepresentation of the study patient population, which could lead to false conclusions.**

There are also a variety of databases available that may contain relevant clinical outcomes data: pharmacy, laboratory, research, and radiology. **Access to all pertinent databases is important for complete understanding of outcome results. It is also critical that the various databases/sources (medical record, survey, and/or administrative data) have the capacity to be linked via a unique patient identification number or other means so that the outcomes data collected is ascribed to the appropriate patient prior to analysis of the data.** As with the medical record and questionnaires, reliability and validity of the information stored in the computerized system is important. One way to check this is to perform a random sample review of the automated records and compare the data elements stored in the computer with the data elements recorded in the "gold standard" manual medical record. Previous work has shown that certain elements, like date of birth, age, dates of certain procedures, and cancer diagnosis and dates are reliably captured in administrative databases, whereas five-year survival status is not (Krousel-Wood et al. 1996b). For selected studies, it may be necessary to pursue a **hybrid methodology** for data collection. This method employs a combination of data sources such as administrative data and medical records data to obtain pertinent clinical information. This approach is accepted by NCQA and others.

Maintaining the confidentiality and security of patient information is critical in all aspects of medical care (Melton 1997). In mental health care, the concern regarding confidentiality and security is magnified because of potential stigma and insurance coverage issues. As a result, access to medical information for mental health patients is often restricted making data collection for outcomes measurement even more challenging. Therefore, careful consideration should be given in planning mental health outcome studies.

Objective 2: Multifaceted Approach to Outcomes Assessment and Performance Improvement

Although outcomes are considered the key component regarding the quality of medical care, it is only one facet of the medical encounter. There are numerous processes (i.e., what we do in medicine) that occur in the delivery of health care. In addition, medical care is given by different providers each with unique qualifications/training and in different settings (e.g., hospital, clinic, emergency room, rural vs. urban areas).

The quality of health care and mental health services has been defined on the basis of three constructs: **outcome, process,** and **structure** (Donabedian 1980; Tarlov 1989; Srebnik et al. 1997). The **outcome** construct has already been addressed in this chapter. The **process** of care construct includes not only the technical aspects of what is done/ordered in the encounter (e.g., antidepressant prescribed, referral to psychiatrists, day treatment therapy initiated) but also the interpersonal style (a subjective measure that may be difficult to quantify feasibly). Most often in outcomes studies and performance improvement activities, the measures that matter outside of the outcomes of interest are the technical components of the process construct: visits (outpatient and emergency room), procedures performed, referrals, medications, tests ordered, expenditures, hospitalizations, coordination and continuity of care (Tarlov 1989). **It is the technical process measures that are closely related to the outcome of interest that are typically reported as surrogate outcomes when the targeted true outcomes are difficult or not feasible to obtain in a timely fashion.**

The **structure** construct includes the characteristics of the health care delivery system, the provider, and the patient. For the most part, the structure characteristics are fixed at the point in time of the medical encounter of interest yet may have a significant impact on the outcome under review. **Understanding the impact of patient characteristics such as age, gender, severity of primary and comorbid conditions, and behavioral risk factors on selected outcomes is key in many outcomes studies and discussions.** For example, if we are assessing outcomes for two recently diagnosed alcoholic female patients in an outpatient setting, we might initially anticipate the five-year survival outcome to be similar provided the treatment regimens prescribed (and hopefully complied with) were the same for both patients. Our assumption would likely be different if we knew that one patient was a twenty-year-old otherwise healthy woman versus a sixty-five-year-old woman with metastatic breast cancer and diabetes. It is important to understand and attempt to quantify factors that can potentially affect outcome measures. These factors can be controlled in the analysis of outcome and performance data, thus allowing more accurate conclusions to be drawn. In a study comparing comorbid illness indices in the assessment of mortality outcome variation for patients undergoing prostatectomy procedures (transurethral [TURP] versus open [OP] approach), we noted the following (Krousel-Wood et al. 1996a): (1) the increased crude mortality associated with TURP versus OP procedures (which was noted by earlier investigators [Roos et al. 1989]) was rendered insignificant once comorbidity was controlled. That is, the increased mortality was associated with patient illness and not type of procedure performed, and (2) not all risk adjustment tools function the same because of differences in components and scoring. Regarding mental health, it is interesting to realize that many risk adjustment tools do not include a component that assesses psychiatric comorbidity. Saravay and Lavin (1994) noted, however, that psychiatric comorbidity contributed to prolonged medical/surgical hospital stays and increased health care utilization post discharge based on a review of twenty-six international and American outcome studies. **Administrators should be aware of the impact of patients' severity of illness in determining the effects of process differences (e.g., type of medications/counseling prescribed) and outcome variation (e.g., suicide attempts/completions) in the care of mental health patients.** Careful consideration should be given to the risk assessment tool selected and the analysis performed on the process and outcome data collected (Iezzoni 1994).

Physician and other provider characteristics are also important when assessing process and outcome information. In particular, the specialty of the physician or other provider may provide insight regarding outcome results. Using depression as an example, primary-care physicians (PCPs) are typically the first contact a depressed patient may have with a medical system. PCP access to and knowledge of appropriate screening and/or counseling techniques, current medical therapies and their effectiveness, relevant and scientifically sound practice guidelines, and/or need for referral to a psychiatric provider for patients with major depression may be limited when compared to a psychiatrist. This could result in differences in outcomes for depressed patients cared for by a PCP versus a psychiatrist (Rost et al. 1998). Efforts targeting minimization of these differences might include implementation of a depression screening tool that is coupled with treatment guidelines and referral mechanisms that PCPs in a busy clinical practice can feasibly use. Rost and others (1998) cautioned that efforts directed at detection of depression without putting processes in place that improve the management of the detected patients may not result in outcome improvement. Care must be taken to address all relevant facets of the structure and process constructs.

A mental health example of the interaction between these constructs is provided in figure 2 using depression as a model. The outcomes listed (functional status and suicide) have been found to be related to the structure and process measures identified. Therefore, changes in one of the structure or process constructs may impact (positively or negatively) the outcomes of interest.

This leads us to the discussion of Continuous Quality Improvement (CQI), now more commonly referred to as Performance Improvement (PI). CQI/PI is an approach to assessing health care that employs methods of industrial quality control to change processes of health care in an effort to optimize health outcomes. Although different models have evolved in industry from the works of Shewhart (1980), Deming (1993), and others, Berwick and others (1990) are usually credited with bringing this approach to health care. In a nutshell the industrial quality control approach utilizes a continuous feedback process that starts with performance monitoring that can identify problems in a delivery system. A multidisciplinary team identifies potential causes of the problems and recommends practice modifications. Once implemented, the practice changes are evaluated and the results of the interventions are assessed. The results can be fed back (often in the form of flow diagrams or charts) to key players in the delivery system. Additional opportunities for improvement of problems can then be identified and the process begins all over again.

The goal of this cyclical process in health care is to improve patient outcomes including satisfaction while focusing on all related medical and system processes. The approach has been successfully utilized in mental health settings as well as other clinical settings (Re and Krousel-Wood 1990).

Examples of CQI in Mental Health

1. A managed care organization employed the tools of CQI to address a problem of access (i.e., long waiting times) for outpatient mental health services from a closed panel of providers during peak demand periods (Keller 1997). Using a multidisciplinary team of physicians, directors, coordinators, and top administrators from the MCO, the access problem was addressed; causes were identified and studied; and solutions were proposed and implemented. Some solutions included establishment of clinical access standards, hiring of a new receptionist, and starting a training program in brief therapy. As a result of the actions taken, average wait times in this selected MCO were significantly reduced from 21.7 days to 6 days

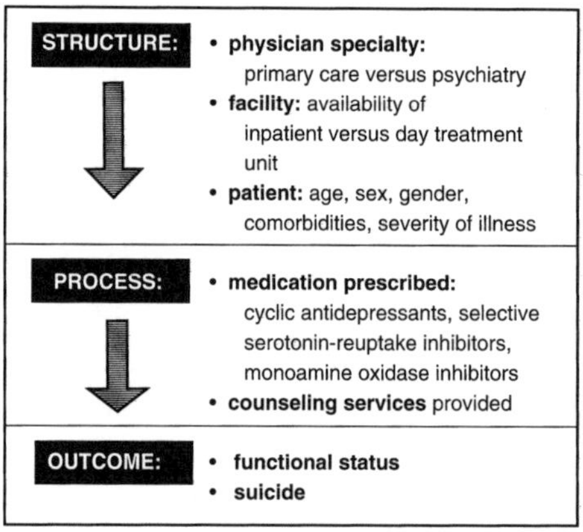

Fig. 2. Construct model for depression

in the nine-month study period; customer satisfaction was improved (Keller 1997).

2. Another application of CQI/PI in the mental health arena was undertaken at an extended-care facility for patients with severe psychiatric illness. The goal of the CQI activity was to improve the Brief Psychiatric Rating Scale (BPRS) administration and presentation and use of findings (Imbornoni et al. 1997). Appropriate use of this objective tool could provide necessary information to enhance clinical assessment and to assess treatment effectiveness over time. Although the tool was already in use by the psychology department, it had not been successfully implemented within the facility. A multidisciplinary team of administrators, psychiatry and rehabilitation personnel, social workers, psychologists, nurses, and information system representatives was formed to identify problems and solutions with the BPRS scale use. A training program for BPRS scale users that addressed potential issues of validity and reliability (among others), was initiated; the authors reported the reliability between the users of the scale increased as a result of this intervention. With the continuous feedback of information to key members of the team as a part of the CQI process, additional opportunities for improvement were identified and solutions implemented: the BPRS evaluation process was standardized; a database was developed; the database output was monitored; and clinical outcomes were measured. The authors concluded that measurement of clinical symptoms and patient outcomes are destined to become critical

determinants in the allocation of increasingly limited health care resources (Imbornoni et al. 1997).

3. Clardy et al. (1998) described the development and implementation of a system for outcomes measurement that incorporated process and outcomes measures for consumers of public health in Arkansas. The project was based on the Shewhart-Deming model of CQI. Although there were some problems noted with voluntary participation in the project, the authors noted that the most significant part of an outcomes management system is the information feedback for CQI (Clardy et al. 1998). **Appropriately timed written and graphical reports that summarize key findings about the patient, processes, and/or outcomes over time can aid decision making for mental health administrators and practitioners.**

4. On a different note, Klegon (1997) described how participating in an accreditation process, like JCAHO, functioned like a performance improvement activity and resulted in an organizational (or network in his example) improvement in performance. An organization's efforts to comply with the accreditation standards often results in identification of areas for improvement. Multidisciplinary teams are useful for identifying and addressing problems in a systematic fashion. Continuous feedback of information to key players and decision makers facilitates the decisions to implement changes in a timely fashion.

5. Another example of a continuous quality improvement/performance activity is the use of the Outcomes Measurement System PsychSentinel, which uses the outcome measure of symptom reduction (Mark and Garet 1997). The number of symptoms at baseline (prior to treatment) is compared to the number of symptoms at follow-up posttreatment; the difference in the scores reveals a range of outcomes from none to complete improvement/reduction in symptoms. Using this system and generating comparative reports provides the information needed to effect change (Mark and Garet 1997). Availability of this and other outcomes data can provide a powerful incentive to effect change (Nathanson 1994).

Criteria for Selecting Topics for Outcomes Study and Performance Improvement Activities

In selecting topics for outcomes study and performance improvement, there are several criteria that can be employed to assist in the decision-making process (table 2). One leading criteria is that the condition or procedure occur frequently in the targeted population. This not only allows for an adequate number of patients that can be studied but also allows for a sufficient number of patients to benefit from treatment or outcome improvements. One way of assessing this in a given population is by using a rank-ordering approach that uses claims data to identify high-volume conditions/procedures (Krousel-Wood et al. 1997). This methodology assesses the frequency of conditions/procedures by way of ICD-9, CPT-4 and/or DRG codes in the claims system(s). The codes are collapsed to the first three digits and the volumes aggregated. Subsequently, the collapsed codes are ranked from highest to lowest, allowing high-volume conditions/procedures to be identified. If details are needed regarding volumes of a specific code (i.e., ICD-9 or CPT-4), the collapsed code can subsequently be broken out into its component codes and their associated frequencies. This approach was employed in a large Southern managed care organization to identify high-volume diagnoses that were relevant to their population. Affective psychosis was identified as one of the top high-volume reasons for admission during the study period. Further analysis revealed that major depression was the leading diagnosis (70 percent) in this collapsed category.

The other criteria are important in identifying areas for further study and may facilitate initiation of an outcomes study or performance improvement activity. Some topics in mental health that fit these criteria include depression, schizophrenia, and substance abuse.

Objective 3: Identify Benefits of and Barriers to Outcomes Assessment and Performance Improvement

There are definite benefits of outcomes assessment and performance improvement in a health care era of apparently diminishing resources. The data and information gathered for these activities result in identification of

TABLE 2. Criteria for Selecting Topics/Conditions for Outcomes Assessment and/or Performance Improvement

- High volume[a]
- High cost[a] (to patient and/or institution)
- Functional impact on patient in terms of morbidity and/or mortality[a]
- Well-defined via clinical endpoints and/or administrative coding
- Medical care can impact natural history of condition[a]
- Quantifiable process and outcomes measures that are linked and relatively feasible to obtain
- Availability of medical evidence regarding treatment effectiveness
- General consensus (among participating parties) regarding treatment approaches and related outcomes
- Potential for improvement in quality of care[a]

[a]See McGlynn and Asch 1998: 14–21.

areas of excellence (also referred to as best practices) and /or areas in need of improvement. Identification of such areas can aid decisions for appropriately directing resources to areas of need. Advances in information systems, outcomes and process measurement tools, and risk assessment methodologies have made engagement in these activities more feasible and productive than in the past. Web site resources (table 3) provide ready access to current information regarding activities and measures available. The use of observational study design techniques in outcome studies allows hypotheses to be generated regarding linkages between process and outcome measures that can be further studied and tested. CQI/PI activities provide a framework for addressing problems identified using quantitative data and a multidisciplinary team approach. In addition, the efforts directed at outcomes measurement and performance improvement provide valuable information regarding efficacy and/or effectiveness of technologies/treatments used today.

Despite the benefits listed, there are a number of barriers to outcomes assessment and performance improvement implementation. Although significant strides have been made in expansion of information systems, development and validation of outcomes and process measurement tools and refinement of risk assessment /adjustment methodologies, there is still much work to be done. In addition, there is a lack of system integration and infrastructure. The ability to link medical systems data (e.g., automated vs. manual medical record data, inpatient with outpatient encounter data, data from different health care organizations) is limited. Inability to track patients longitudinally across health care providers and episodes of care is another barrier. Privacy and confidentiality regarding

TABLE 3. Web Site Resources for Outcomes and Performance Improvement Activities and Measures in Mental Health

Web Site Address	Description
www.aahp.org	American Association of Health Plans
www.ahcpr.gov	Agency for Health Care Policy and Research
www.facct.org	Foundation for Accountability in Healthcare
www.hcfa.gov	Health Care Financing Administration
www.jcaho.org	Joint Commission on Accreditation of Healthcare Organizations
www.ncqa.org	National Commission for Quality Assurance
www.nih.gov	National Institutes of Health
www.nimh.gov	National Institutes of Mental Health
www.outcomes-trust.org	Medical Outcomes Trust
www.phc4.org	Pennsylvania Health Care Cost Containment Council

use of data continue to be issues that must be adequately addressed. There are also costs associated with outcomes and performance improvement project setup and implementation that administrators often find difficult to address in the face of economic hardships. Lastly, practitioners and administrators may be indifferent, resistant to change and/or wary of punitive action as a result of involvement in these activities (Joint Commission 1994). Nevertheless, participation in these activities will likely be the norm for all mental health administrators and practitioners in the near future.

Conclusion

Outcome and performance data, if appropriately collected and used, are measures that matter in health care. Assessing and addressing the links between outcome and performance are the key to maximizing quality of medical care. The number of generic and disease-specific tools developed to date as well as the availability of computerized information systems and CQI/PI techniques provide the necessary components for a foundation in outcomes assessment and performance improvement. Although participation in outcomes assessment and performance improvement activities add to the complexity of mental health administration and practice, the information derived from these efforts will facilitate decision making that will lead to optimization of outcomes in a cost-efficient manner for patients with mental health disorders.

GLOSSARY

Benchmark Best practices that institutions/organizations/groups can strive toward or exceed with respect to outcomes and process measures

Clinical performance indicator A measure that assesses whether the appropriate process of care was provided in the right time frame for selected patient(s) with a given medical condition(s) (e.g., the percentage of patients with major depression who received an antidepressant within an appropriate time frame)

Clinical practice guidelines Recommendations/statements for providers regarding appropriate treatment processes for selected medical conditions. Other similar terms include practice parameters, algorithms, treatment guidelines

Comorbid conditions Other disease condition(s) a patient has in addition to the primary disease under study or review. These conditions can potentially impact the relevant processes and outcomes of care

CQI/PI Continuous quality improvement or performance improvement: activities that employ methods of industrial quality control to change processes of health care in an effort to maximize health outcomes

Effectiveness A measure of how well a treatment works under usual circumstances in a general population

Efficacy A measure of how well a treatment works under ideal circumstances in a targeted patient population

FACCT Foundation for Accountability, a not-for-profit organization that brings together consumer groups and purchasers with the goal of helping Americans make better decisions in health care

HEDIS Health Plan Employer Data Information Set was codeveloped by NCQA and representatives of employers and health plans. It includes indicators for mental health and substance abuse

Hybrid methodology A method of data collection that uses a combination of data sources to obtain the value of the measure of interest. A commonly used hybrid methodology is the use of administrative data and medical record data

JCAHO Joint Commission on Accreditation of Healthcare Organizations, a not-for-profit organization that accredits health care entities

NCQA National Committee for Quality Assurance, a not-for-profit organization that accredits managed care organizations

Outcomes A measure of the end result of what happens to patients as a consequence of their encounter(s) with the health care system; a construct of quality that reflects functional status, clinical endpoints, satisfaction, and/or cost

Process A construct of quality that reflects what is done/ordered/prescribed in the medical care of patients

Reliability The extent to which the results of a measurement are reproducible or repeatable on subsequent trials

Structure A construct of quality that reflects the patient, provider, and system characteristics

Surrogate outcome Process measure that is closely related to the outcome of interest and serves as a proxy for the outcome

Validity The extent to which a tool truly measures what it intends to measure

REFERENCES

Berwick, D. M., A. B. Godfrey, and J. Roessner. 1990. *Curing Healthcare: New Strategies for Quality Improvement.* San Francisco: Jossey-Bass Publishers.

Chowanec, G. D. 1994. Continuous quality improvement: Conceptual foundation and application to mental health care. *Hospital and Community Psychiatry* 45:789–93.

Chowanec, G. D. 1996. The fall and rise of TQM at a public mental health hospital. *Journal on Quality Improvement* 22:19–26.

Clardy, J. A., et al. 1998. Implementing a statewide outcomes management system for consumers of public mental health services. *Psychiatric Services* 49:191–95.

Codman, E. A. 1914. The product of a hospital. *Surg Gynecol Obstet* 18:491–96.

Deming, W. E. 1993. *The New Economics for Industry, Education, Government.* Cambridge, MA: Institute of Technology, Center for Advanced Engineering Study.

Donabedian, A. 1980. *Explorations in Quality Assessment and Monitoring.* Vol. 1: *The Definition of Quality and Approaches to Its Assessment.* Ann Arbor, MI: Health Administration Press.

Epstein, A. 1995. Sounding board: Performance reports on quality—prototypes, problems and prospects. *New England Journal of Medicine* 333: 57–61.

Gordis, L. 1996. *Epidemiology.* Philadelphia: W. B. Saunders Company.

Hannan, E. L., et al. 1997. Using medical claims data to assess provider quality for CABG surgery: Does it work well enough? *Health Services Research* 31:659–78.

HEDIS 3.0. 1998. *Technical Specifications.* Vol. 2: *1999.* National Committee for Quality Assurance.

Iezzoni, L. I., ed. 1994. *Risk Adjustment for Measuring Health Care Outcomes.* Ann Arbor, MI: Health Administration Press.

Imbornoni, S., et al. 1997. Objective measurement of psychiatric symptoms: A quality improvement process for inpatient care. *Journal on Quality Improvement* 23:183–95.

Joint Commission. 1994. *A Guide to Establishing Programs for Assessing Outcomes in Clinical Settings.* Oakbrook Terrace, IL: Joint Commission on Accreditation of Healthcare Organizations.

Joint Commission. 1996. *Comprehensive Accreditation Manual for Health Care Networks.* Oakbrook Terrace, IL: Joint Commission on Accreditation of Healthcare Organizations.

Joint Commission. 1997. *National Library of Healthcare Indicators, Health Plan and Network Edition.* Oakbrook Terrace, IL: Joint Commission on Accreditation of Healthcare Organizations.

Keller, G. A. 1997. Management for quality: Continuous quality improvement to increase access to outpatient mental health services. *Psychiatric Services* 48:821–25.

Klegon, D. A. 1997. JCAHO mental health care network accreditation as a performance improvement project. *Psychiatric Services* 48:359–63.

Krousel-Wood, M. A., et al. 1996a. Comparison of three different comorbid illness indices in the assessment of outcomes: The case of prostatectomy. *Journal of General Internal Medicine* 11:32–38.

Krousel-Wood, M. A., et al. 1996b. The National Clinics Research Consortium's (NCRC) use of administrative databases for collaborative study: The case of prostatectomy. *American Journal of Managed Care* 2:269–75.

Krousel-Wood, M.A., et al. 1997. Technology utilization in United States health facilities. Abstract presented at the Thirteenth Annual International Society of Technology Assessment in Healthcare, Barcelona, Spain.

McDowell, I., and C. Newel. 1987. *Measuring Health: A Guide to Rating Scales and Questionnaires.* New York: Oxford University Press.

McGlynn, E. A., and S. M. Asch. 1998. Developing a clinical performance measure. *American Journal of Preventive Medicine* 14:14–21.

Mark, H., and D. E. Garet. 1997. Interpreting profiling data in behavioral health care for a continuous quality improvement cycle. *Journal on Quality Improvement* 23:521–28.

Melton, L. J. 1997. Sounding board: The threat to medical records research. *New England Journal of Medicine* 337:1466–70.

Nathanson, P. 1994. Influencing physician practice patterns. *Top Health Care Finance* 20:16–25.

NCQA Standards for Accreditation of Managed Behavioral Healthcare Organizations. 1998. Washington, DC: NCQA Publications Center.

NCQA Standards for Accreditation of Managed Care Organizations. 1998. Washington, DC: NCQA Publications Center.

Norquist, G. S., and K. M. MaGruder. 1998. Views from funding agencies: National Institute of Mental Health. *Medical Care* 36:1306–8.

Re, R. N., and M. A. Krousel-Wood. 1990. How to use continuous quality improvement theory and statistical quality control tools in a multispecialty clinic. *Quality Review Bulletin* 16:391–97.

Roos, N. P., et al. 1989. Morality and reoperation after open and transurethral resection of the prostate for benign prostatic hyperplasia. *New England Journal of Medicine* 320:1120–24.

Rost, K., et al. 1994. The deliberate misdiagnosis of major depression in primary care. *Archives of Family Medicine* 3:333–37.

Rost, K., et al. 1998. Persistently poor outcomes of undetected major depression in primary care. *General Hospital Psychiatry* 20:12–20.

Rothman, K. J. 1986. *Modern Epidemiology.* Boston: Little, Brown.

Saravay, S. M., and M. Lavin. 1994. Psychiatric comorbidity and length of stay in the general hospital. *Psychosomatics* 35:233–52.

Shewhart, W. A. 1980 [1931]. *Economic Control of Quality of Manufactured Product.* Milwaukee: ASQ Quality Press.

Srebnik, D., et al. 1997. Development of outcome indicators for monitoring the quality of public mental health care. *Psychiatric Services* 48:903–9.

Tarlov, A. R., et al. 1989. The medical outcomes study. An application of methods for monitoring the results of medical care. *Journal of the American Medical Association* 262:925–30.

Wennberg, J. E., ed. 1998. *Dartmouth Atlas of Health Care.* Chicago: American Hospital Publishing.

About the Authors

Kenneth Gaver, M.D.

Most of Kenneth Gaver's career has been dedicated to mental health administration. He has been chief executive officer of the state Departments of Mental Health and Mental Retardation in Oregon, Ohio, and Texas and medical director of two private psychiatric hospitals and a national psychiatric hospital company. For over twenty years he represented psychiatric hospitals on numerous councils, committees, and JCAHO task forces, and he has provided consultation to many public and private mental health and psychiatric institutions. He is a past president of both the National Association of State Mental Health Program Directors and the National Association of Private Psychiatric Hospitals.

Marshall B. Kapp, J.D., M.P.H.

Marshall Kapp was educated at Johns Hopkins University (B.A.), George Washington University School of Law (J.D., with Honors), and Harvard University School of Public Health (M.P.H.). He is the Frederick A. White Professor of Service in the Departments of Community Health and Psychiatry at Wright State University School of Medicine, where he is also director of the Office of Geriatric Medicine and Gerontology. He holds an adjunct faculty appointment at the University of Dayton School of Law and is admitted to practice law in Florida and before numerous federal courts. During 1998–99 he was the Dr. Arthur Grayson Memorial Distinguished Visiting Professor of Law and Medicine at Southern Illinois University.

Marie A. Krousel-Wood, M.D., M.S.P.H.

A board-certified preventive medicine specialist, Dr. Krousel-Wood received her M.D. degree (1987) from Louisiana State University School of Medicine and her M.S.P.H. degree (1991) from the Tulane University School of Public Health and Tropical Medicine, where she was inducted into the Delta Omega Honor Society for public health. Dr. Krousel-Wood is a staff scientist in the Outcomes Assessment Department of the research division at Alton Ochsner Medical Foundation and serves as the director of outcomes measurement for Ochsner Health Plan. She is a member of the faculty at Tulane University School of Public Health and Tropical Medicine and associate professor of family and community medicine at Tulane University School of Medicine, and she is co-investigator on a project funded by the Department of Defense entitled "The Role of Technology in Reducing Healthcare Costs."

William F. Martin, Psy.D., M.P.H., M.A.
William "Marty" Martin is currently clinical assistant professor in the Department of Health Systems Management at Tulane University School of Public Health and Tropical Medicine. Prior to joining the Tulane faculty, Dr. Martin served as director of Workforce Diversity at the Johns Hopkins Hospital. In addition, Dr. Martin has assisted numerous organizations as an employee and consultant in the areas of EAP design, human resources development, mental health benefits design, organization development, performance management, training, and worksite wellness. Dr. Martin is a licensed clinical psychologist, a member of the National Register of Health Service Providers in Psychology, and a certified health education specialist.

Douglas Mossman, M.D.
Douglas Mossman graduated from Oberlin College (B.A.) and the University of Michigan Medical School (M.D.) and completed his psychiatry residency at the University of Cincinnati College of Medicine. He is professor and director of the Division of Forensic Psychiatry at Wright State University and is a member of the adjunct faculty at the University of Dayton School of Law.

Ray G. Newman, Ph.D., CPA
Ray Newman joined Tulane University in March 1995 as vice chancellor for administration and finance at the Tulane University Medical Center. He also holds an appointment of clinical associate professor in the Department of Health Systems Management at Tulane University's School of Public Health and Tropical Medicine. In addition to teaching, he provides program direction and serves as advisor for medical students enrolled in the joint MD/MPH degree program. Dr. Newman earned his Ph.D. and Master of Philosophy degrees at New York University, where his major areas of study were finance and health policy. He also holds an M.B.A. degree from California State University and a B.S. degree from East Central University. Dr. Newman is a CPA, a Fellow in the American College of Healthcare Executives, and a Fellow in the Healthcare Financial Management Association. His background includes experience in operations, consulting, and education.

Raymond F. Patterson, M.D.
A graduate of Northwestern University (1973) and Howard University School of Medicine (1977), Raymond Patterson has had extensive experience as an administrator and director of forensic, clinical, and mental health organizations and as a consultant to numerous correctional, educational, hospital, professional, and law enforcement organizations. He is a surveyor for the Joint Commission on Accreditation of Healthcare Organizations. From 1987 until 1992 he served as forensic services administrator, Commission on Mental Health Services, for the District of Columbia. Dr. Patterson has consistently maintained a private practice in general and forensic psychiatry in Washington, DC, and he has been appointed to the School of Medicine Faculties at Howard University, the University of Maryland, and Georgetown University. He is the recipient of many awards from professional organizations, associations, and agencies, including the U.S. Department of Justice, the U.S. Secret Service, hospitals, and patient rights groups.

Birge D. Reichard, Ph.D.
Birge Reichard is president of Berkeley Developmental Resources, Inc., a consulting company that provides services in the areas of organization behavior, organization development, and human resources. He consults with senior managers in business and health care organizations in the United States, Canada, and the United Kingdom. Formerly an associate professor of organization behavior at the American University in Washington, DC, Dr. Reichard has been a manager in human resources for Bell System and Xerox Canada and served as vice president and professional director of the NTL Institute for Applied Behavioral Science. As a psychologist, he previously collaborated with Dr. Rodenhauser as a coauthor of *The Small Group Trainer's Survival Guide* (1992)—a guide to risk prevention and management in affective education.

Paul Rodenhauser, M.D.
Paul Rodenhauser is professor of psychiatry, director of medical student education in psychiatry, and assistant dean for academic and counseling services at Tulane University School of Medicine, and adjunct professor, health systems management and international health and development, at Tulane University School of Public Health and Tropical Medicine. He is a 1963 graduate of Jefferson Medical College of Thomas Jefferson University, where he was elected to Alpha Omega Alpha his junior year. His experiences in residency education in psychiatry at The Sheppard and Enoch Pratt Hospital, which included serving as chief resident, inspired interest in administration and education. He is president of the American Association of Psychiatric Administrators.

Charles L. Scott, M.D.
Board certified in general, child and adolescent, forensic, and addiction psychiatry, Charles Scott is director of forensic psychiatry training and an assistant professor of psychiatry at the University of California, Davis. Dr. Scott is an instructor for the National Forensic Psychiatry Board Review Course and has lectured nationally on mental health law for hospital administrators. Dr. Scott has served as a clinical consultant to jails, prisons, and maximum-security forensic psychiatric units. He has published chapters related to child psychiatry and juvenile dangerousness and has coauthored chapters on legal issues related to the psychiatric assessment of dangerousness.

R. Dennis Staton, Ph.D., M.D.
Dennis Staton holds S.B. and S.M. degrees from MIT (1960, 1961), a Ph.D. degree in Medical Science from Harvard University (1969), and an M.D. degree from the University of Miami School of Medicine (1973). He completed psychiatric residency training at the University of Vermont in 1977. Currently he serves as a board-certified psychiatrist at Lakeland Mental Health Center in Moorhead, Minnesota, and as a child and adolescent psychiatric consultant in Fargo, North Dakota. His twenty-year career in academic psychiatry includes professorships at Albany Medical College and the University of North Dakota School of Medicine, where he also served as director of UND's psychiatric residency training program for ten years. He has authored or coauthored approximately forty-five published articles.

E. Gordon Whyte, Ph.D.

Gordon Whyte has held leadership positions in both the public and the private sectors, including not-for-profit and proprietary hospitals, community mental health centers, social service agencies, and skilled nursing facilities. He holds an M.H.A. and a Ph.D. degree in health care administration with a specialty in health care marketing as well as degrees in counseling and psychology. He is a licensed nursing home administrator and the vice chairman of the Department of Health Systems Management at Tulane University School of Public Health and Tropical Medicine. Dr. Whyte's marketing work has been nationally recognized by the Academy of Health Services Marketing of the American Marketing Association.

Index

Bold page numbers indicate glossary definitions.

Accounts receivable ratio, 173, **175**
Accounts receivables, 153, **175**
Accreditation, 41, **49**
Accrual accounting, 149, **175**
Acid test ratio, 167, **175**
Activity ratios, 173
Adverse selection, 22, **25**
Advertising, 68, **73**
Affirmative action, 223, **229**
Age Discrimination in Employment Act (ADEA), 222
Alternative dispute resolution (ADR) programs, 227
Americans with Disabilities Act (ADA), 82, **97**
 and documentation, 130
Arbitration, 227, **229**
Assets, 150, **175**
Assisted suicide, 114
Association of Medical Superintendents of American Institutions for the Insane, 78, **97**
Asylum, 78, **97**
Average payment period, 174, **175**

Bad debts, 153, **175**
Balanced Budget Act, 17
Balance sheet, 149, **176**
Bargaining unit, 227, **229**
Basic earning power (BEP) ratio, 170, **176**
Behavioral Health Care Corporation (BHCC), 46, **49**
Behavioral Health Care Organization (BHO), 33, 46, **49**
Benchmark, 239, **250**
Benefits, 220
Break-even analysis, 159, 176

Capitation, 19
 full-risk capitation, 23
 partial-risk capitation, 22
Capitation payment, 16, **25**
Career paths, 207, **229**
Carve-out, **49,** 83, **97**
Carve-out programs, 47
Cash accounting, 149, **176**
Cash flow statement, 155
Casualty, 130, **144**
Change in organizations, 189, 191, 192, **198**
Charity care, 12
Civil commitment, 107
Civilian Health and Medical Program for the Uniformed Services (CHAMPUS), 38, 43, **49**
Clinical performance indicator, 234, **250**
Clinical Practice Guidelines, 237, **250**
Commission on Accreditation of Rehabilitation Facilities (CARF), 41, **49,** 85, 91, **97**
Common law, 128, **145**
Community Mental Health Centers Act, 39, 81, **97**

Community mental health programs, 39
Comorbid conditions, 242, **250**
Comorbidity, 35, **49**
Competence, 130, 137, **145**
Competitive advantage, 202
Comprehensive Accreditation Manual for Hospitals, The, 90, **97**
Confidentiality, 115, **124, 145**
  and assessment, 242
  and documentation, 140
  and outcomes, 249
  and situations that supercede, 141
Conflict management, 185
Conflict of interest, 23
Consultation-liaison services, 34
Consumer behavior, 54, **73**
Continuous quality improvement or performance improvement (CQI/PI), 245, **251**
Corporatization of health care delivery, 5
  effect of, 6
  quality of care, 7
Correctional facilities, 43
Cost reduction, 20
Cost shifting, 12, 15, **25**
Credit, 149, **176**
Current asset activity ratio, 173, **176**
Current assets, 150, **176**
Current liabilities, 151, **176**
Current ratio, 166, **176**
Cutoff score, 208, **229**

Damages, 103, **124**
Dangerousness, 105
Debit, 149, **176**
Debt management, 171
Debt ratio, 172, **176**
Deemed status, 92, **97**
Defamation, 140, **145**
Demographic segmentation, 64, **73**
Depreciation, 154, **176**
Differentiation, 71, **73**
Direction setting, 182, **198**
Direct selling, 69, **73**
Discipline, 225, **229**
Discounted payments, 6, **26**
Discretionary costs, 4, **26**
Documentation guidelines, 132
Double-entry accounting, 148, **176**
Due process, 226, **230**

Effectiveness, 236, **251**
Efficacy, 236, **251**
Elastic demand, 4, **26**
Emancipated minor, 119, **125**
Emergency rooms, 33
Employee Retirement Income Security Act (ERISA), 24, 117, **125**
Employment and labor laws, 221
Equity theory, 220, **230**
Exempt, 218, **230**

Federal qualification, 47, **49**
Feedback, 205, 212, 214, 216, **230**
Fiduciary relationship, 130, **145**
Fiduciary responsibility, 6, **26**
Financial ratio analysis, 165, **176**
First in–first out (FIFO), 153, **176**
Fixed asset activity ratio, 173, **177**
Fixed charge coverage ratio, 172, **177**
Fixed costs, 158, **177**
Focus group, 59, **73**
Foundation for Accountability (FACCT), 237, **251**
Full-risk capitation, 23, **26**
Fund balance, 152, 154, **177**
Funding sources, 81, 83, **97**

Golden handcuffs, 218, **230**
Governing body, 83, **97**
Grievance, 226, **230**
Guardian *ad litem,* 120, **125**

Health care costs, 2
  and consumers, 5
  and employers, 2, 13
  and Medicaid, 3
  and Medicare, 2, 17

Health Care Financing Administration (HCFA), 12, 84, 85, 92, **97**
and Quality Improvement System for Managed Care (QISMC), 239
Health care free market, 11
Health Maintenance Organization (HMO), 8, 33, 46, **49,** 85, **98**
Health Plan Employer Data Information Set (HEDIS), 238, 239, **251**
Helpful mechanisms in organizations, 188, **198**
Historical costs, 152
Human resources functions, 205
Hybrid methodology, 242, **251**

Income statement, 154, **177**
Indemnity insurance, 7, 8, **26**
Independent practice association (IPA), 33, 46, **50**
Informed consent, 109, **125**
and documentation, 137
Insanity, 78, **98**
Integrated insurance-delivery systems, 8
Intentional torts, 102, 110, **125**
Inventories, 153, **177**
Inventory turnover, 173, **177**

Job grade, 218, **230**
Job posting and bidding, 207, **230**
Joint Commission on Accreditation of Healthcare Organizations (JCAHO), 35, **50,** 85, 90, **98,** 129, 139, 238, **251**
and documentation, 129, 139

Kirkbride, Thomas, 79

Labor market, 220, **230**
Labor relations, 227, **230**
Last in–first out (LIFO), 154, **177**
Leadership, 188, **198**
Leadership tasks, 188
Lewin, Kurt, 179, 191
Liabilities, 151, **177**
Long-term assets, 151, **177**
Long-term liabilities, 151, **177**
Lunatic, 77, **98**

Mainstreaming, 47, **50**
Malpractice, 102, 103, **145**
and documentation, 129
and suicide, 104
Managed behavioral health care organization (MBHCO), 47, **50**
Managed care, 8, 54
and legal liability, 117
and outcomes measurement, 237
Managed care organization (MCO), 15, 45, **50,** 91, **98,** 238
and performance improvement (PI), 238
Managers of services, 84, **98**
Managing organization change, 191
first-order organization change, 191
second-order organization change, 191
Market demand, 63, 65
Market forecast, 62, **73**
Marketing, 55, **73**
Marketing information and research, 56
Marketing information system (MrkIS), 57
Marketing mix, 66, **73**
Marketing orientation, 55, **74**
Market segmentation, 63
Mature minor, 119, **125**
Measurements of quality, 87, **98**
Mediation, 227, **230**
Medicaid, 92, **98**
and documentation, 129
and managed care, 48
Medicaid 1115 waiver, 40, **50**
Medicaid 1915B waiver, 40, **50**
Medical director, 39
Medical evidence, 129, 136
Medical-loss ratio, 7, **26**
Medical Outcomes Trust, 240
Medical records, 240

Medicare, 92, **98**
  and documentation, 129
Medicare certification, 37, **50**
Mental health care benefits, 16
Mental health care costs, 3
Mental Health Parity Act, 17
Mental health service delivery systems
  basic structure, 83
  historical context, 77
Merit-based pay, 219, **230**
Military hospitals, 42
Minor, 119, **125**
Mission, 86, **98**
Multiple specialty groups, 33

National Alliance for the Mentally Ill (NAMI), 85, **98**
National Association of Psychiatric Health Systems (NAPHS), 16, 36, **50**
National Association of State Mental Health Program Directors (NASMHPD), 38, **50**
National Commission on Correctional Health Care (NCCHC), 85, 92, **98**
National Committee for Quality Assurance (NCQA), 41, **50,** 85, 91, **98,** 238, **251**
National Council on Patient Information and Education (NCPIE), 138
National Institutes for Occupational Safety and Health, 222
Needs assessment, 61, 76, **98**
Negligence, 102, **125,** 136
Net book value, 153, **177**
Not-for-profit delivery systems, 10
Numbers of days cash on hand ratio, 167, **177**

Oligopolistic management, 10, **26**
Operating earnings before interest and taxes (EBIT), 170
Operating margin ratio, 170, **177**
Organization, 180, **198**
Organizational development, 211, **230**
Organization diagnosis, 189, **198**
Organization purpose, 180
Organization structure, 183
Orientation, 210, **230**
Outcome assessment drivers, 236
Outcomes, 234, 243, **251**
  and medical records, 240
Outpatient commitment, 108
Owner's equity, 151, **177**

Parens patriae, 107, **125,** 143, **145**
Parity coverage for mental illness, 17
Partial risk capitation, 22, **26**
Patients' access to records, 139
Pay-for-performance plans, 219, **231**
Performance improvement (PI), 245, **251**
Performance management, 182
Performance management system, 182, 214
Physician decision making, 24
Point of service (POS) plans, 46, 54, **50**
Police power, 107
Positioning, **74,** 202
Positioning the organization, 70
Preferred provider organization (PPO), 33, 46, **50,** 85, **99**
Price earnings ratio, 174, **178**
Price sensitive, 4, **27**
Prima facie, 141, **145**
Primary demand, 66, **74**
"Principles of Practice," 79, **99**
Prison Litigation Reform Act (PLRA), 82, **98**
Privacy Act, 139, **145**
Private practice, 32
Private psychiatric hospitals, 35
  and revenues, 37
Privatization, 10, **26**
Privilege, 115, **125**
Process, 235, 238, 243, **251**
Process notes, 135, **145**
Professional autonomy, 25
Professional certification, 85, **99**
Profitability ratios, 167

Profit margin ratio, 170, **178**
Progressive discipline, 226, **230**
Progress notes, 133, **145**
Promotional strategies, 68
Prospective payment, 6, **26**
Provider panel, 33, **50**
Providers of services, 83, **99**
Provider-sponsored organizations, 9, **26**
Psychiatric units in general hospitals, 35
Psychographic segmentation, 64, **74**
Publicity, 69, **74**

Randomized controlled trials, 236
Rationing medical care, 25
Recipients of services, 83, 85, 86, **99**
Recognition, 216, **230**
Recruitment, 206, **230**
Refreezing, 193, **198**
Regulatory agencies, 85
  basic principles, 88
  common characteristics, 89
  mission and intent, 86
  review preparation, 93
Regulatory standards, 87, **99**
Reinforcement, 187, **198**
Relationship marketing, 68
Relationships, 185, **198**
Reliability, 240, **251**
Res ipsa loquitur, 104, **125**
Resistance to change, 195, **198**
Restraints, 79, 81, **99**
Retrospective cost-based reimbursement, 6, **26**
Return on assets (ROA) ratio, 171, **178**
Return on equity (ROE) ratio, 171, **178**
Rewards, 187, **199,** 216, **231**
Rights of minors, 119
  and involuntary hospitalization, 108
Right to die, 113
Right to refuse treatment, 112
Right to treatment, 111
Risk adjustment, 22, **26**
Risk pool, 47, **51**
Risk selection, 22, **26**
Risk shifting, 15, **26**

Scatter beds, 34, **51**
Seclusion, 79, 81, **99**
Segmentation, 63, **74**
Selection, 208, **231**
Selective demand, 65, **74**
Sexual harassment , 222, **231**
Shadow buying, 15, **26**
Socialization, 205, 207, **231**
Social Security Disability Insurance (SSDI), 130
Spoliation of evidence, 128, **145**
Stakeholders, 83, **99**
Standard of proof, 103
Standards for Accreditation of Managed Behavioral Healthcare Organizations, 47
Standards for Accreditation of Managed Care Organizations, 91, **99**
Standards for Health Services in Jails, 92, **99**
Standards Manual for Organizations Serving People with Disabilities, 91, **99**
State mental health agencies, 18
State Mental Health Authority (SMHA), 38, 40, **51**
State mental hospitals, 38
Statement of cash flows, 155, **178**
Statute of limitations, 137, **145**
Statutory or legal requirements, 88, **99**
Strict liability, 102, **125**
Structure, **199,** 243, **251**
Subpoena, 143, **145**
Surrogate outcome, 235, **251**
SWOT analysis, 203

Tarasoff duty, 142, **145**
Targeting, 65, **74**
Testimonial privilege, 115, 143, **145**
Therapeutic privilege, 110, **125**

Times interest earned (TIE) ratio, **178,** 182
Tort, 102, **125**
Tort law, 102
Training, 210, **231**

Unfreezing, 191, **199**
Unions, 227
Utilization management (UM), 46, **51**

Validity, 241, **252**
Variable costs, 158, **178**
Vertical integration, 9, **26**
Veterans Affairs Medical Centers, 41

Wage, 218, **231**
Weisbord's Six Box Model, 181
Withholding, 47, **51**
Withholds, 16, **26**
Work group, 182, **199**